Corneal Dystrophies

Developments in Ophthalmology

Vol. 48

Series Editor

F. Bandello Milan

Corneal Dystrophies

Volume Editors

Walter Lisch Hanau
Berthold Seitz Homburg/Saar

43 figures, 30 in color, and 13 tables, 2011

KARGER

Basel · Freiburg · Paris · London · New York · New Delhi · Bangkok · Beijing · Tokyo · Kuala Lumpur · Singapore · Sydney

Walter Lisch
Department of Ophthalmology
City Hospital of Hanau
Leimenstrasse 20
DE - 63450 Hanau (Germany)

Berthold Seitz
Department of Ophthalmology
University of Saarland
Kirrbergerstrasse 1, Building 22
DE - 66424 Homburg/Saar (Germany)

Library of Congress Cataloging-in-Publication Data

Corneal dystrophies / volume editors, Walter Lisch, Berthold Seitz.
p. ; cm. -- (Developments in ophthalmology, ISSN 0250-3751 ; v. 48)
Includes bibliographical references and indexes.
ISBN 978-3-8055-9720-3 (hard cover : alk. paper) -- ISBN 978-3-8055-9721-0 (electronic ed.)
1. Cornea -- Diseases -- Genetic aspects. I. Lisch, W. (Walter) II. Seitz, Berthold. III. Series: Developments in ophthalmology ; v. 48. 0250-3751
[DNLM: 1. Corneal Dystrophies, Hereditary. W1 DE998NG v.48 2011 / WW 220]
RE336.C6624 2011
617.7'19 -- dc22

2011006820

Bibliographic Indices. This publication is listed in bibliographic services, including Current Contents® and Index Medicus.

www.karger.com
Printed in Switzerland on acid-free and non-aging paper (ISO 9706) by Reinhardt Druck, Basel
ISSN 0250–3751
ISBN 978–3–8055–9720–3
e-ISBN 978–3–8055–9721–0

Contents

List of Contributors

Anthony J. Aldave
The Jules Stein Eye Institute
David Geffen School of Medicine
The University of California
100 Stein Plaza, Los Angeles, CA 90095 (USA)
E-Mail aldave@jsei.ucla.edu

Satoshi Kawasaki
Department of Ophthalmology
Kyoto Prefectural University of Medicine
465 Kajii-cho, Hirokoji-agaru
Kawaramachi-dori, Kamigyo-ku
Kyoto 602-0841 (Japan)
E-Mail bluenova@koto.kpu-m.ac.jp

Arbi J. Khemichian
Kresge Eye Institute
Wayne State University School of Medicine
4717 St Antoine, Detroit, MI 48201 (USA)
E-Mail arbi.khemichian@utsouthwestern.edu

Shigeru Kinoshita
Department of Ophthalmology
Kyoto Prefectural University of Medicine
465 Kajii-cho, Hirokoji-agaru
Kawaramachi-dori, Kamigyo-ku
Kyoto 602-0841 (Japan)
E-Mail shigeruk@ophth.kpu-m.ac.jp

Walter Lisch
Department of Ophthalmology
City Hospital of Hanau
Leimenstrasse 20, DE - 63450 Hanau (Germany)
E-Mail lisch.hanau@t-online.de

H.U. Møller
Department of Pediatric Ophthalmology
Viborg Hospital
DK - 8800 Viborg (Denmark)
E-Mail hans.ulrik.moeller@sygehusviborg.dk

Somasheila I. Murthy
Cornea and Anterior Segment Service
L. V. Prasad Eye Institute
Kallam Anji Reddy Campus,
L. V. Prasad Marg, Banjara Hills,
Hyderabad, 500 034 (India)
E-Mail smurthy@lvpei.org

Varsha M. Rathi
Cornea and Anterior Segment Service
L. V. Prasad Eye Institute
Kallam Anji Reddy Campus,
L. V. Prasad Marg, Banjara Hills,
Hyderabad, 500 034 (India)
E-Mail varsharathi@lvpei.org

Berthold Seitz
Department of Ophthalmology
University of Saarland
Kirrbergerstrasse 1, Building 22,
DE - 66424 Homburg/Saar (Germany)
E-Mail berthold.seitz@uks.eu

Geeta K. Vemuganti
School of Medical Sciences
University of Hyderabad
Hyderabad, 500046 (India)
E-Mail gkvemuganti@gmail.com

Jayne S. Weiss
Chair of Department of Ophthalmology
Herbert Kaufman, Professor of Ophthalmology
Louisiana State University Health Science
Center
2020 Gravier Street
New Orleans, LA 70112 (USA)
E-Mail jayneweiss@aol.com

Preface

The cornea, basically composed of the epithelium, stroma and endothelium, is the major refractive organ of the optic system in addition to serving as a mechanical barrier. The corneal epithelium is the most regular arrangement of stratified epithelium in the whole human body. The cells, composed of 6–7 different layers, are tightly and orderly arranged without intercellular spaces. We know that some corneal dystrophies are only characterized by the occurrence of epithelial opacities. The contact lens-induced regression of opacities in epithelial corneal dystrophies can be interpreted as a contact lens-induced reduction of epithelial layers. As in other connective tissues, the major portion of the corneal stroma is composed of extracellular matrix macromolecules which are responsible for the strength and transparency of this tissue. Some corneal dystrophies are thought to result in part from abnormalities in corneal stromal cell function. Corneal stromal cells synthesize and degrade matrix materials during corneal morphogenesis and proper metabolism of such materials is essential. Stromal corneal dystrophies recur after decades on the graft due to the long-term transformation of transplant keratocytes into pathological host keratocytes. The corneal endothelium is a monolayer of hexagonal cells that forms the posterior corneal surface. An intact monolayer of endothelial cells is essential for the functional endothelial barrier to preserve a relative dehydration of the stroma and a prerequisite to corneal transparency. If the integrity of the monolayer is breached, corneal edema rapidly develops as we can see in some endothelial corneal dystrophies. The replacement of the posterior cornea, called Descemet's stripping endothelial keratoplasty, represents a modern and sophisticated surgical procedure in the treatment of endothelial corneal dystrophies.

With the revolution in molecular genetics, our understanding of corneal dystrophies has changed in the last 15 years as disorders have been mapped and the genes responsible have been identified. Today we know that phenotypic heterogeneity – the same gene causing different forms of corneal dystrophies – and genotypic heterogeneity – different genes causing a phenotypically identical corneal dystrophy – do exist. Research continues to uncover important knowledge on corneal dystrophies. However, the identification of the gene and mutations in corneal dystrophies can only be interpreted as a start in the mosaic puzzle for uncovering the complex relationships in the pathophysiological molecular mechanisms. In general, further molecular physiological examinations and the evaluation of animal models are necessary to precisely define the essential protein defect in the different types of corneal dystrophy. The development of a causal therapy for corneal dystrophies must be the big scientific challenge in the future.

Walter Lisch, Hanau
Berthold Seitz, Homburg/Saar

Lisch W, Seitz B (eds): Corneal Dystrophies.
Dev Ophthalmol. Basel, Karger, 2011, vol 48, pp 1–8

IC3D Classification of Corneal Dystrophies

H.U. Møller[a] · Jayne S. Weiss[b]

[a]Department of Pediatric Ophthalmology, Viborg Hospital, Viborg, Denmark; [b]Department of Ophthalmology, Louisiana State University Health Science Center, New Orleans, La., USA

Abstract

The International Committee for Classification of Corneal Dystrophies (IC3D) has provided an update of our knowledge on corneal dystrophies. This chapter gives the summary of clinical findings, onset, course, genetics, nosology, light and electron microscopy as well as immunohistochemistry for 25 different entities included as corneal dystrophies in this survey. A category number from 1 through 4 is assigned, reflecting the level of evidence supporting the existence of a given dystrophy.

Myths and Misconceptions

Most of the original papers on classic corneal dystrophies were published in German: lattice corneal dystrophy [1–3], granular corneal dystrophy and macular corneal dystrophy [4], Fuchs corneal dystrophy [5], Reis-Bücklers corneal dystrophy [6, 7], Schnyder corneal dystrophy [8], Meesmann corneal dystrophy [9], posterior polymorphous corneal dystrophy [10] and Thiel-Behnke corneal dystrophy [11]. Although the German scientific language provided a precise as well as detailed description of what the first author observed, unfortunately, because of language barriers, few ophthalmologists outside central Europe were actually able to read the original papers. Nevertheless, numerous authors from the past and present who write about dystrophies still quote these original dystrophy publications despite the fact that these same authors have never read the original articles.

As a result, over the decades, the accuracy of the information attributed to the original article tends to become diluted by inexact summaries of the seminal article or translations of a questionable quality. Furthermore, many ophthalmologists continue to use quotations of their predecessors even though they have never read their papers. This behavior has led to the incorporation of numerous mistakes in peer-reviewed publications which get repeated again and again until ultimately they are accepted as facts. One example of this phenomenon is that in publications in the 1960s using the newly invented electron microscope 'the ring like structure' on the slit lamp of Reis-Bücklers corneal dystrophy was described [12].

Time has demonstrated that there is no such finding on examination of Reis-Bücklers corneal dystrophy. Most probably this error occurred because there was confusion with Bücklers' description in his 1938 thesis [13] of what we currently call granular corneal dystrophy type 2, in which small rings of granules are often found.

In those days, the medical world and the spectrum of differential diagnoses were quite different. For example, Wehrli [14–17] published almost 100 pages in 1905 and 1906 arguing that granular corneal dystrophy was due to tuberculosis. Perhaps he was right as his patients could have had tuberculosis – as well. Many patients in that era probably had scarring and neovascularization resulting from infections that are rarely seen today. Consequently, this older literature is not easy to read and to interpret today.

Furthermore, it is important for the reader of the 21st century to understand that the papers from 50 or even 100 years ago were written in quite a different scientific world. A professor ranking high in the ophthalmological hierarchy was not easily contradicted. Peer-reviewed journals with strict rules for critical review of a scientific paper before it was accepted to the journal did not exist. As a consequence, unsubstantiated statements and actual errors were published and then often repeated in subsequent papers.

In addition, today many ophthalmologists continue to find the subject of corneal dystrophies difficult because of the rarity of many of these entities. Due to the *founder effect,* dystrophies are often unevenly distributed geographically. It is likely that there are no ophthalmologists that can claim they have examined many patients with each of the corneal dystrophies. Thus, there is no such person as *a corneal dystrophy expert* with expertise in the entire field. As a consequence, even many authors of book chapters in renowned textbooks have copied mistakes from their predecessors.

Finally, the nomenclature of some of the corneal dystrophies is misleading and has led to misdiagnosis of patients. The name 'Schnyder crystalline corneal dystrophy' suggests that corneal crystalline deposition is an integral part of this disease. However, only 50% of patients with Schnyder crystalline corneal dystrophy have corneal crystals. Numerous patients with Schnyder crystalline corneal dystrophy without crystals have escaped correct diagnosis for decades precisely because the nomenclature is confusing [18].

In 2005, at the World Cornea Congress, it was clear that it was time to address this issue in order to finally revise the nomenclature. One of the authors (J.S.W.) asked the other members of the Board of Directors of the Cornea Society to lend their support for this idea of the creation of an international committee to revise the corneal dystrophy nomenclature. The goal was to recruit an international panel of

Table 1. The panel of the IC3D

Jayne S. Weiss (Chair)
H.U. Møller
Walter Lisch
Shigeru Kinoshita
Anthony J. Aldave
Michael W. Belin (Vice-Chair)
Tero Kivelä
Massimo Busin
Francis L. Munier
Berthold Seitz
John Sutphin
Cecilie Bredrup
Mark J. Mannis
Christopher J. Rapuano
Gabriel Van Rij
Eung Kweon Kim
Gordon K. Klintworth
Rasik Vajpayee
Tony Bron (Consultant)

ophthalmologists, geneticists and ophthalmic pathologists with firsthand experience with the clinical, genetic, and histopathologic findings of all the corneal dystrophies. With these experts, we could critically evaluate the literature and remove outdated or incorrect information [19].

There is no absolute truth in medicine and the 2008 IC3D classification shall probably be followed by another classification in due course; but at present this paper hopefully is a useful guideline for better understanding of corneal dystrophies. The full text can be retrieved on the website www.corneasociety.org/ic3d.

The Panel of IC3D

The panel of the committee comprised a group of interested world experts (table 1). Most of the participants of the group had 1 or 2 corneal dystrophies in which they had a special interest. The advantage of the diversity of the committee was that many different scientific traditions were present. Some were splitters and found it important to subdivide all entities to the smallest possible details, while others were pragmatic lumpers wanting a classification easily useable to the general ophthalmologist. Fruitful discussions ended in the compromise presented below; the paper is the result of days of discussions and thousands of e-mails over a period of 4 years.

The Classification

A classification is the systematic arrangement of similar entities on the basis of certain differing characteristics. The IC3D classification includes most of the diseases usually named corneal dystrophies (table 2).

Our first challenge was whether or not the word dystrophy should be discarded and substituted by the term 'genetic corneal diseases'. This approach was supported by the fact that there is no universally accepted definition for a corneal dystrophy [20]. However, despite the nebulous meaning, 'corneal dystrophy' is still the name universally accepted in textbooks. Consequently, the compromise was to continue to use this name. The term corneal dystrophy was first utilized almost 100 years ago when Fuchs used the word for the disease still having his name attached as an eponym. He postulated that dystrophic tissues resulted from lack of nourishment, hormones, blood, and nerve supply [5]. Why the word 'dystrophic' has been attached to entities later proven to be genetic is not known, and is probably just a coincidence. But genetics is the key for understanding these diseases, and the recent availability of genetic analyses has demonstrated the shortcomings of the phenotypic method of corneal dystrophy classification [19].

The dystrophies are typically classified by the level of the cornea that is involved, which separates these entities into epithelial and subepithelial, Bowman layer, stromal, Descemet membrane, and endothelial dystrophies. This distinction is partly obsolete, but kept to be true to tradition.

Four Categories

In the new classification system, all corneal dystrophies have been categorized into 4 levels:

- category 1: a well-defined corneal dystrophy in which the gene has been mapped and identified and specific mutations are known;
- category 2: a well-defined corneal dystrophy that has been mapped to 1 or more specific chromosomal loci, but the gene(s) remain(s) to be identified;
- category 3: a well-defined corneal dystrophy in which the disorder has not yet been mapped to a chromosomal locus;
- category 4: this category is reserved for a suspected new, or previously documented, corneal dystrophy, although the evidence for it, being a distinct entity, is not yet convincing.

The category assigned to a specific corneal dystrophy can be expected to change over time as knowledge progressively advances. Eventually, all valid corneal dystrophies should attain the level of category 1; macular corneal dystrophy is an example of a category 1 dystrophy. Conversely, over time and with further information, some entities that are category 4 may be shown not to be distinct entities and may be removed [19].

Table 2. The IC3D classification – name, abbreviations, Mendelian Inheritance in Man (MIM) number (http://www.ncbi.nlm.nih.gov/sites/entrez), and category

Name	IC3D abbreviation	MIM no.	Category
Epithelial basement membrane dystrophy	EBMD	121820	1
Epithelial recurrent erosion dystrophy	ERED	122400	3, 4
Subepithelial mucinous corneal dystrophy	SMCD	None	4
Meesmann corneal dystrophy	MECD	122100	1
Lisch epithelial corneal dystrophy	LECD	none	2
Gelatinous drop-like corneal dystrophy	GDLD	204870	1
Reis-Bücklers corneal dystrophy	RBCD	608470	1
Thiel-Behnke corneal dystrophy	TBCD	602082	1
Grayson-Wilbrandt corneal dystrophy	GWCD	none	4
Classic lattice corneal dystrophy	LCD1	122200	1
Lattice corneal dystrophy, Meretoja type	LCD2	105120	1
Granular corneal dystrophy 1	GCD1	121900	1
Granular corneal dystrophy 2	GCD2	607541	1
Macular corneal dystrophy	MCD	217800	1
Schnyder corneal dystrophy	SCD	121800	1
Congenital stromal corneal dystrophy	CSCD	610048	1
Fleck corneal dystrophy	FCD	121850	1
Posterior amorphous corneal dystrophy	PACD	none	3
Central cloudy dystrophy of François	CCDF	217600	4
Pre-Descemet corneal dystrophy	PDCD	none	4
Fuchs endothelial corneal dystrophy	FECD	136800	1, 2 or 3
Posterior polymorphous corneal dystrophy	PPCD	122000	1 or 2
Congenital hereditary endothelial dystrophy 1	CHED1	121700	2
Congenital hereditary endothelial dystrophy 2	CHED2	217700	1
X-linked endothelial corneal dystrophy	XECD	none	2

Naming of the Specific Entities

Most of the corneal dystrophies have been published under very different names in the past, and the panel found that universally accepted names are a key point for communication in future literature. In this survey, names of all the dystrophies have been chosen among many options considering both a long-standing tradition and which name was the commonly used one – and the classification system has also been adopted by Online Mendelian Inheritance in Man (OMIM) (http://www.ncbi.nlm.nih.gov/sites/entrez).

One example of the difficulties with the former nomenclature system is lattice corneal dystrophy, which has had as many as 3 eponyms attached: Biber-Haab-Dimmer [1–3]. Many types and varieties of lattice corneal dystrophy have been published (table 3). The panel chose to lump these as 'classic lattice corneal dystrophy and varieties'. The Meretoja type is actually not a corneal dystrophy but a hereditary systemic

Table 3. Lattice corneal dystrophy (classic) and varieties

Lattice types I–VII
Lattice types IIIA and IIIB
Lattice intermediate types I and IIIA
Lattice late-onset type
Lattice deep stromal
Lattice atypical
Lattice Meretoja type – a recessive entity

Table 4. Templates give clinical information of the entities described in the classification

Name/alternative names/eponyms
Gene
Gene locus
Signs
Symptoms
Onset
Course
Light microscopy
Electron microscopy
Confocal microscopy
Category
Key references
MIM No.
Inheritance

amyloidosis; however, it is included in the classification as it could be mistaken for one of the lattice varieties. The classification system is meant to be malleable and be able to change with increasing knowledge. The future shall probably reveal phenotype-genotype correlations of many different mutations, and some later classification will determine whether this lumping of lattice corneal dystrophy subtypes was the correct decision. It is likely that a phenotyping of corneal dystrophies – as well as many other genetic eye diseases – will describe that different mutations have distinct clinical signs and symptoms, and later probably modifier genes will appear and explain some of the not yet understood clinical diversities.

The Templates of the Classification

Templates comprising clinical information describe each disease (table 4) and the text is accompanied by 60 color pictures to give the reader an introduction when browsing for a diagnosis. Key references are provided, as well as the OMIM number (http://www.ncbi.nlm.nih.gov/sites/entrez) for a quick link to further clinical information.

All members of the panel wrote up templates of diseases of their special interest, and all templates were later peer reviewed by 2 other members of the committee and scrutinized through discussions at meetings of the panel to minimize mistakes.

The Use of the Classification in the Peer Review Process When Publishing New Findings

It is the hope of the committee that ophthalmologists will adopt a more scientific approach to the field of genetic corneal disease by both detailed characterization of phenotypic changes and obtaining genetic testing when indicated. The IC3D nomenclature classification should effectively endorse more scientific and objective criteria for determining whether a 'new' corneal dystrophy or dystrophy variant has indeed been discovered. Hopefully authors and reviewers alike will be more stringent before the publication of these entities [19].

Conclusion

In 2008, the IC3D devised a new classification system for the corneal dystrophies which included genetic, clinical and histopathologic information as well as slit lamp photos of 25 corneal dystrophies. This new system is user-friendly and upgradeable and can be retrieved on the website www.corneasociety.org/ic3d [19].

References

1 Biber H: Ueber einige seltene Hornhauterkrankungen: die oberflächliche gittrige Keratitis, inaugural dissertation, Zürich, 1890.

2 Haab O: Die gittrige Keratitis. Zeitschr Augenheilkd 1899;2:246.

3 Dimmer F: Ueber oberflächliche gittrige Hornhauttrübung. Zeitschr Augenheilkd 1899;2: 354–361.

4 Groenouw A: Knötchenförmige Hornhauttrübungen (Noduli corneae). Arch Augenheilkd 1890;21: 281–289.

5 Fuchs E: Dystrophia epithelialis corneae. Graefes Arch Clin Exp Ophthalmol 1910;76:478–508.

6 Reis W: Familiäre, fleckige Hornhautentartung. Dtsch Med Wochenschr 1917;43:575.

7 Bücklers M: Über eine weitere familiäre Hornhaut-Dystrophie (Reis). Klin Monatsbl Augenkeilkd 1949;114:386–397.

8 Schnyder W: Mitteilung über einen neuen Typus von familiärer Hornhauterkrankung. Schweiz Med Wschr 1929;10:559–571.

9 Meesmann A: Über eine bisher nicht beschriebene dominant vererbte Dystrophia epithelialis corneae. Ber Zusammenkunft Dtsch Ophthalmol Ges 1938; 52:154–158.

10 Schlichting H: Blasen- und dellenförmige Endotheldystrophie der Hornhaut. Klin Monatsbl Augenkeilkd 1941;107:425–435.

11 Thiel HJ, Behnke H: Eine bisher unbekannte subepitheliale hereditäre Hornhautdystrophie. Klin Monatsbl Augenheilkd 1967;150:862–874.

12 Grayson M, Wilbrandt H: Dystrophy of the anterior limiting membrane of the cornea. Am J Ophthalmol 1966;61:345–349.
13 Bücklers M: Die erblichen Hornhautdystrophien. Klin Monatsbl Augenheilkd 1938;3:48–55.
14 Wehrli E: Die knötchenförmige Hornhauttrübung (Groenouw) eine primäre, isolierte, chronische, tuberkulöse Erkrankung der vorderen Schichten der Cornea - Lupus corneae. Z Augenheilk 1905;13: 322–334.
15 Wehrli E: Die knötchenförmige Hornhauttrübung (Groenouw), eine primäre, isolierte, chronische, tuberkulöse Erkrankung der vorderen Schichten der Cornea - Lupus corneae. Z Augenheilk 1905;13: 461–478.
16 Wehrli E: Die knötchenförmige Hornhauttrübung (Groenouw) eine primäre, isolierte, chronische, tuberkulöse Erkrankung der vorderen Schichten der Cornea - Lupus corneae. Z Augenheilk 1905;13: 558–578.
17 Wehrli E: Weitere klinische und histologische Untersuchungen über den unter dem Bilde der knötchenförmigen Hornhauttrübung (Groenouw) - chronischen verlaufenden lupus. Arch Augenheilk 1906;55:126–184.
18 Weiss JS: Visual morbidity in thirty-four families with Schnyder crystalline corneal dystrophy (an American Ophthalmological Society thesis). Trans Am Ophthalmol Soc 2007;105:616–648.
19 Weiss JS, Møller HU, Lisch W, et al: IC3D classification of the corneal dystrophies. Cornea 2008; 27(suppl 2):S1–S83.
20 Warburg M, Møller HU: Dystrophy: a revised definition. J Med Genet 1989;26:769–771.

H.U. Møller, PhD
Department of Pediatric Ophthalmology, Viborg Hospital
DK–8800 Viborg (Denmark)
Tel. +45 7844 5551, E-Mail hans.ulrik.moeller@viborg.rm.dk

Lisch W, Seitz B (eds): Corneal Dystrophies.
Dev Ophthalmol. Basel, Karger, 2011, vol 48, pp 9–23

The Clinical Landmarks of Corneal Dystrophies

Walter Lisch[a] · Berthold Seitz[b]

[a]Department of Ophthalmology, City Hospital of Hanau, Hanau, and [b]Department of Ophthalmology, University of Saarland, Homburg/Saar, Germany

Abstract

The International Committee for Classification of Corneal Dystrophies, briefly IC3D, was founded to develop a new, internationally accepted classification of corneal dystrophies (CDs) based on modern clinical, histological and genetical knowledge. Being members of the IC3D, the authors of this chapter present a clinical landmark survey of the different CDs. The ophthalmologist is the first to examine and to diagnose a new patient with a probable CD using a slit lamp. The presented landmarks are supposed to be a bridge for the ophthalmologists to precisely define the corneal opacities of a presumed CD. This bridge makes it easier for them to study the IC3D publication and to get more information including adequate differential diagnosis.

The ophthalmologist is the first to examine and diagnose a new patient with a probable corneal dystrophy (CD) using a slit lamp [1]. We agree with Wiggs [2] that genotypes need phenotypes.

Before slit lamp examination, the ophthalmologist should ask the patient if there is a family history of visual impairment or corneal disease. Then the patient should be asked about systemic and skin disorders, such as rosacea or atopy. At the same time, a macroscopic examination of the facial skin and the lids is very important concerning the evaluation of dry skin, of altered red and thin scale-like skin, of the appearance of facial telangiectasias, and of altered thickened lid margins.

Additionally, the patient has to be asked about unstable visual impairment. A very important question concerns recurrent pain with red eyes and epiphora. A patient with various forms of CD can present pseudoinflammatory signs and be misdiagnosed as having acute keratitis. Bilateral or alternating ocular pain, red eye and epiphora in such a situation are not the result of a bacterial or viral infection but of CD-induced recurrent erosions.

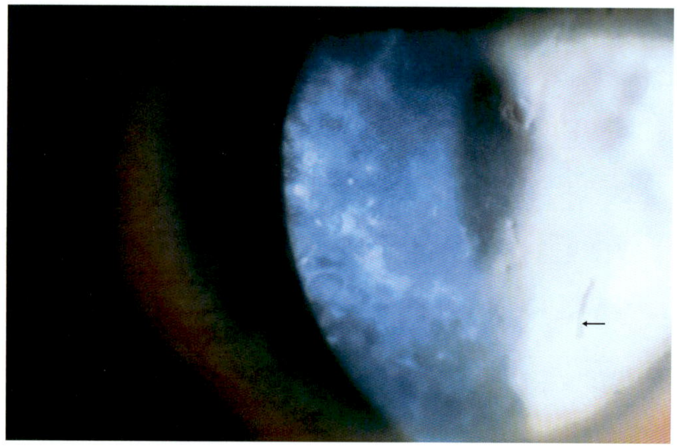

Fig. 1. Large diffuse, subepithelial opacification simulating keratitis but masking lattice corneal dystrophy. One lattice line (arrow).

CD-specific diffuse opacities, often combined with pain due to additional epithelial erosion, can be misdiagnosed as bacterial infiltration of the cornea with the consequence of a completely inadequate therapy (fig. 1). Therefore, it is a must to examine the contralateral cornea directly and indirectly with dilated pupil. The occurrence of contralateral corneal opacities can be a hint to a CD and exclude an inflammatory process.

Johann Wolfgang von Goethe once said: 'What's hardest of all? It's what you think is easiest: to see with your eyes what's before your eyes.' In line with this general wisdom from Goethe, the ophthalmologist, too, always has a differential diagnostic challenge of an ophthalmological disease.

The slit lamp examination in general, but especially of patients with a CD, must be performed according to precise rules as outlined below.

1 Examination of both eyes.
2 Examination with dilated pupils in direct and indirect (retro) illumination.
3 Topographical determination of the corneal opacification with regard to the layer:
   - superficial
   - stromal
   - endothelial
   - combination
4 Characteristic opacity pattern in direct illumination. The opacity pattern represents the CD-specific opacity. Example: central disk fig. 2).
5 Characteristic opacity units in direct and indirect illumination. The opacity units form the opacity pattern, often best seen in indirect illumination. Example: solitary clear microcysts in Meesmann CD (fig. 3a).
6 So-called pseudoinflammatory signs due to a CD (fig. 1).

In what follows, the differential diagnosis of typical opacity patterns and units in CD [3] will be described.

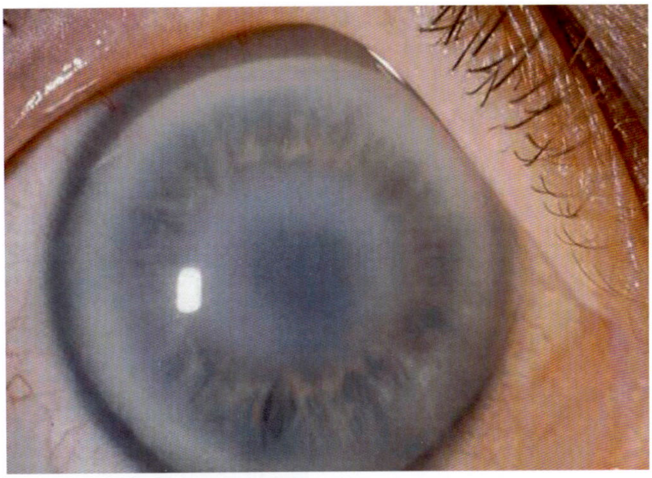

Fig. 2. Central, subepithelial diffuse disk of Schnyder corneal dystrophy in direct illumination; arcus lipoides.

Clear Cyst-Like Opacities

a Meesmann CD: directly – diffuse, grayish epithelial opacities in different patterns; indirectly – solitary, clear microcysts (fig. 3a).
b Lisch epithelial CD: directly – diffuse, grayish epithelial opacities in different patterns; indirectly – crowded, clear microcysts (fig. 3b).
c Bron's bleb-like type of epithelial basement membrane dystrophy (EBMD): directly – not visible; indirectly – subtle, clear cyst-like units (solitary or crowed) at the level of epithelium (fig. 3c).
d Fabry disease represents a systemic X-linked disease [4] disclosing directly – diffuse, grayish epithelial opacities in form of 'cornea verticillata' – and indirectly – crowded, punctifom (no cysts!) units and forming whorled lines (fig. 3d).

Line-Like Opacities

a Map-like type of EBMD [5]: directly and indirectly – irregular, epithelial lines with areas of grayish haziness, above all in the central part of the cornea (fig. 4a).
b Fingerprint-like type of EBMD: directly, but better indirectly – above all paracentral epithelial, fine, curvilinear and parallel lines (fig. 4b).
c Hypertrophic nerves: directly and indirectly, several conditions feature enlarged corneal nerves. The most important is multiple endocrine neoplasia type 2B.
d Fabry disease: directly and indirectly – epithelial, whorled lines consisting of crowded punctiform units (fig. 3d).
e Lattice lines of lattice corneal dystrophy (LCD) and variants: directly – network of delicate, branching lattice-like lines that occur in the anterior stroma paracentrally;

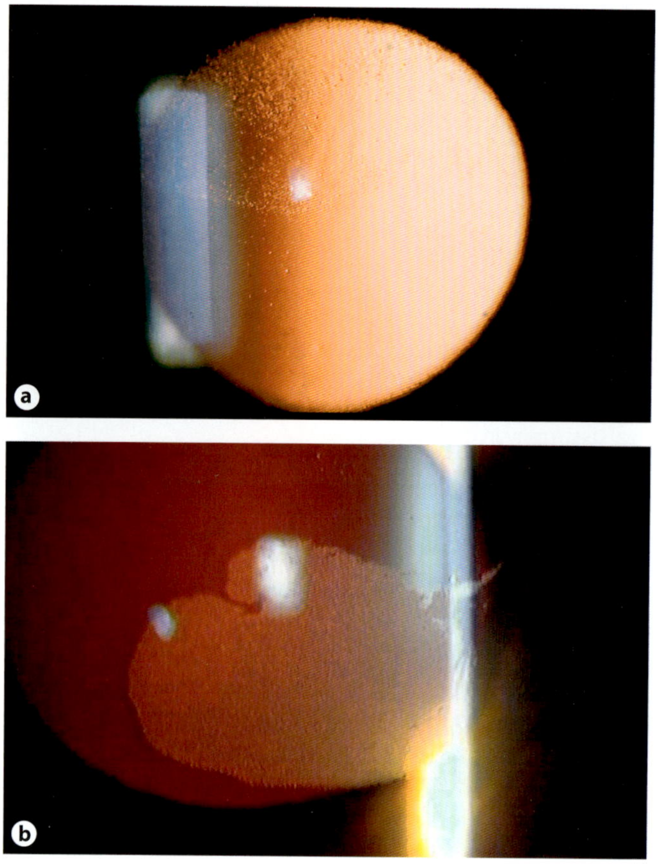

Fig. 3. **a** Solitary, clear microcysts in Meesmann CD in indirect illumination. **b** Crowded, clear microcysts in Lisch epithelial CD in indirect illumination (courtesy of S. Butros).

indirectly – lattice lines are refractile with a double contour (fig. 4c, d). LCD type 2, a misnomer for the Meretoja syndrome, represents an autosomal dominantly inherited systemic amyloidosis with similar corneal lattice lines as in LCD and variants [6].

f Haab's striae (congenital glaucoma): directly and indirectly – breaks in Descemet's membrane in form of single or multiple, elliptical, glassy, parallel ridges on the posterior cornea either peripherally or centrally.

g Scars of Descemet's membrane after corneal hydrops.

Fleck-Like Opacities

a Cogan's dot-like type of EBMD: directly and indirectly – irregular round, oval, ameboid or putty-gray opacities, mostly in the center of corneal epithelium (fig. 5a).

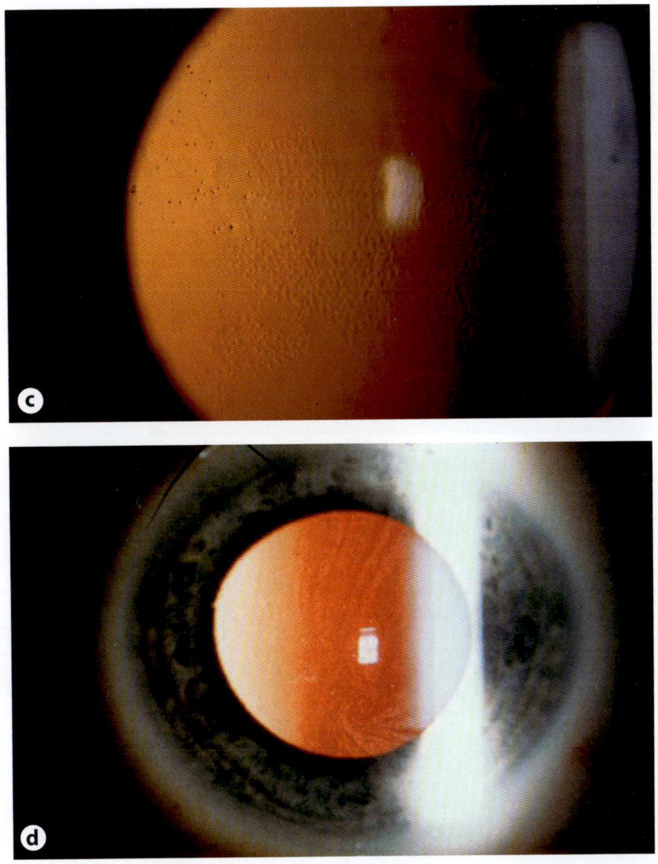

Fig. 3. **c** Bron's clear blebs in EBMD in indirect illumination. **d** Fabry disease: crowded, punctiform (no cysts) units forming whorled lines in indirect illumination.

b Granules of granular corneal dystrophy type 1 (GCD1): directly and indirectly – multiple small crumb-like granules, separated from one another in the center of the anterior corneal stroma (fig. 5b).

c Stars and rings of GCD2 [7]: directly and indirectly – rings with punched out centers and powdery disks or stellate elements, all located in the center of anterior corneal stroma (fig. 5c).

d Flecks of macular corneal dystrophy: directly and indirectly – flecks through the whole cornea and diffuse stromal ground-glass haze (fig. 5d).

e Nodular-like type of gelatinous drop-like corneal dystrophy: directly and indirectly – whitish-yellow nodular lesions (mulberry-like) in the center of subepithelial cornea (fig. 5e).

f Prominent nodular lesions of Salzmann's degeneration: directly and indirectly – whitish prominent nodular lesions paracentrally at the level of the anterior cornea.

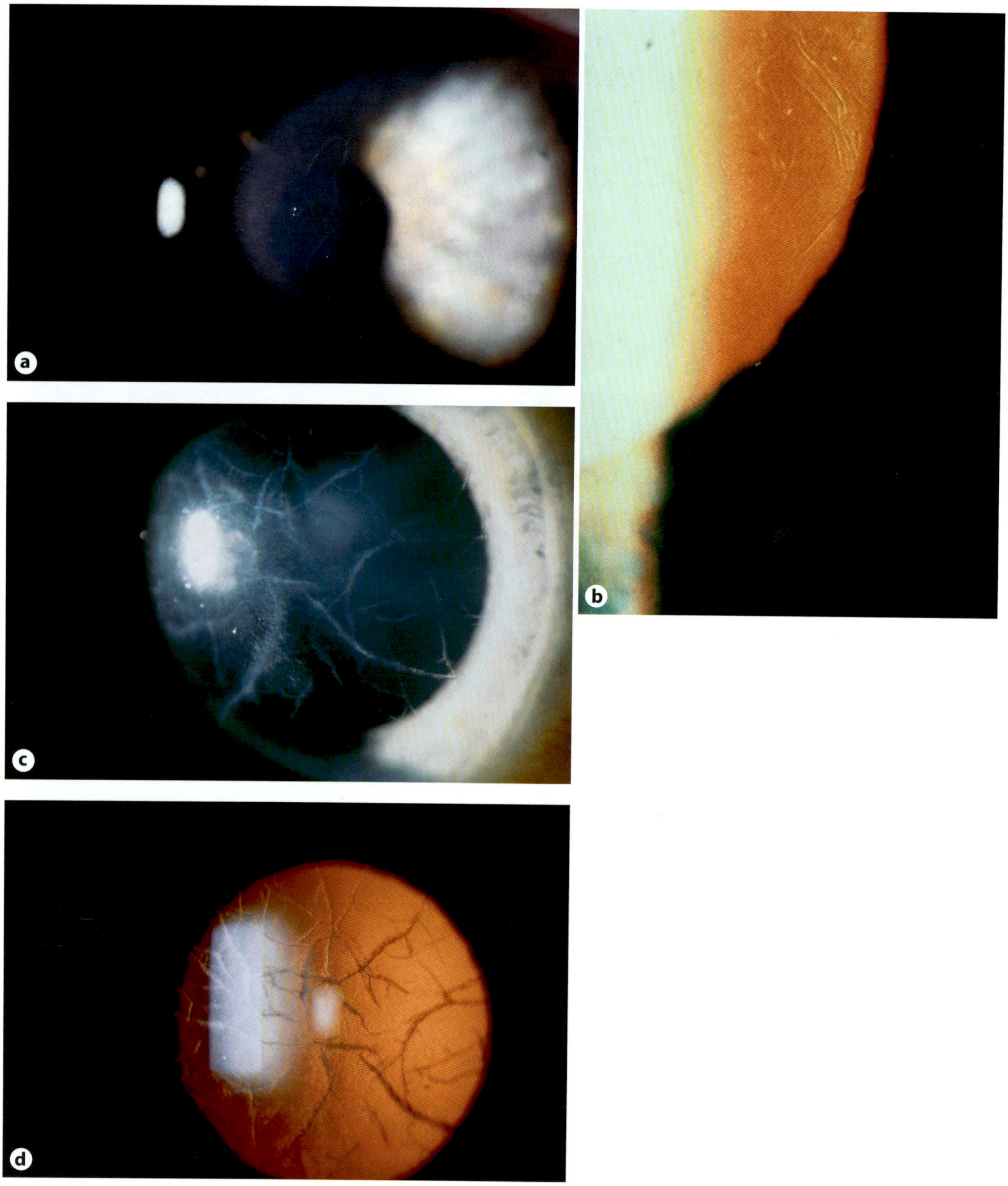

Fig. 4. **a** Map-like opacities of EBMD in direct illumination. **b** Fingerprint-like opacities of EBMD in indirect illumination. **c** Lattice lines of LCD in direct illumination. **d** Refractile, lattice lines with a double contour of LCD in indirect illumination.

Unique Opacities

a Geographic-like opacity of Reis-Bücklers corneal dystrophy [8]: directly and indirectly – subepithelial, geographic-like pattern (fig. 5f).
b Honeycomb-like opacity of Thiel-Behnke corneal dystrophy [9]: directly and indirectly – subepithelial, honeycomb-like pattern (fig. 6a).
c Dense reticular-like opacity of homozygous GCD2 [10]: directly and indirectly – subepithelial, dense reticular gray-white opacities with several round translucent spaces (fig. 6b).

Crystalline-Like Opacities

a Crystals in Schnyder corneal dystrophy [11]: directly and indirectly – subepithelial central disk- or ring-like opacity consisting of crowded, multicolored, needle-shaped crystals (fig. 6c); often associated with arcus lipoides.
b Crystals in Bietti's crystalline dystrophy: directly and indirectly – subepithelial peripheral corneal and retinal crystals.
c Crystals in cystinosis: directly and indirectly – solitary, punctiform, multicolored crystals throughout the whole stroma.
d Crystals in monoclonal gammopathy (monoclonal gammopathy of undetermined significance and malign form) [12]: directly and indirectly – solitary, punctiform, multicolored crystals throughout the stroma, often combined with patch-like or diffuse opacities (fig. 6d).

Anterior Band-Like Opacities

a Secondary band keratopathy in congenital hereditary endothelial dystrophy (CHED) types 1 and 2: rare; indirectly (dilated pupil) – above and below the band diffuse stromal or endothelial changes.
b Secondary band keratopathy in posterior polymorphous corneal dystrophy (PPCD): rare; indirectly (dilated pupil) – above and below the band diffuse stromal or endothelial changes.
c Secondary band keratopathy in X-linked endothelial corneal dystrophy (XECD) [13] (fig. 6e): only in male patients; indirectly (dilated pupil) – above and below the band moon-crater-like endothelial changes.
d Band keratopathy in gelatinous drop-like corneal dystrophy: directly and indirectly – anterior band keratopathy seems to be the most prevalent of this dystrophy. It is unclear if band keratopathy represents a transition to mulberry-like opacity.

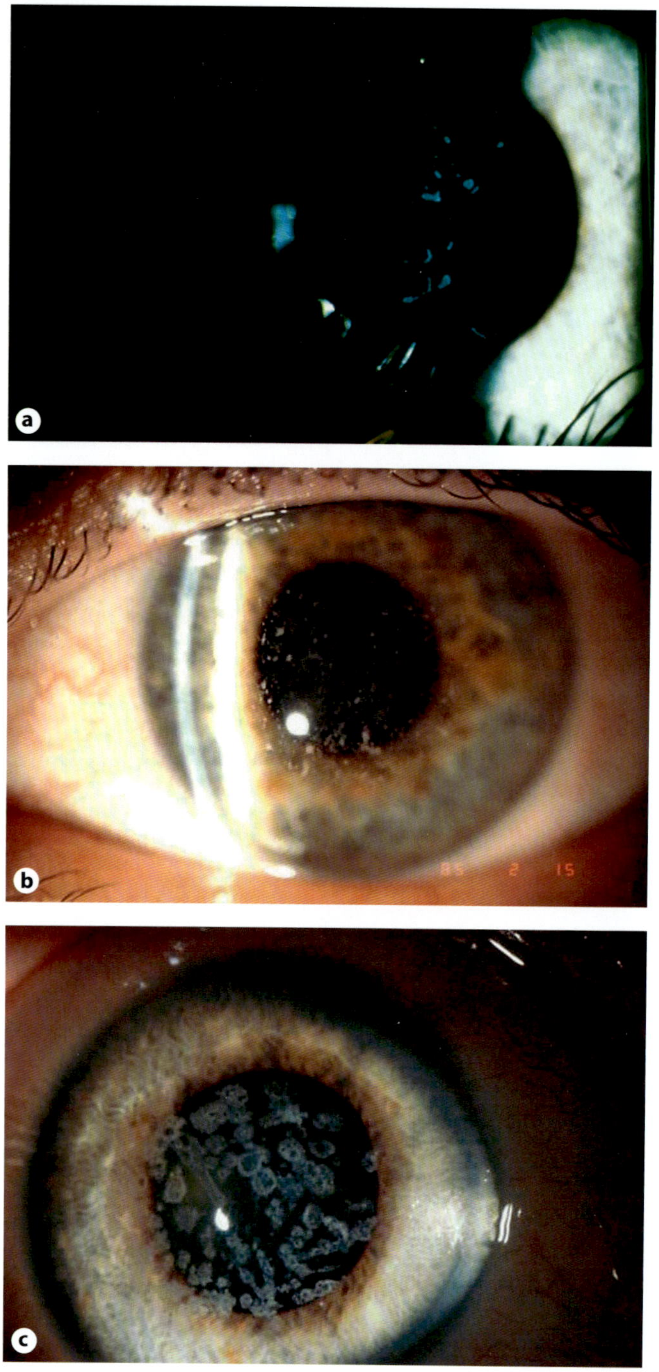

Fig. 5. **a** Cogan's dots of EBMD in direct illumination. **b** Multiple, central granules of GCD1 in direct illumination. **c** Central stars and rings of GCD2 in direct illumination.

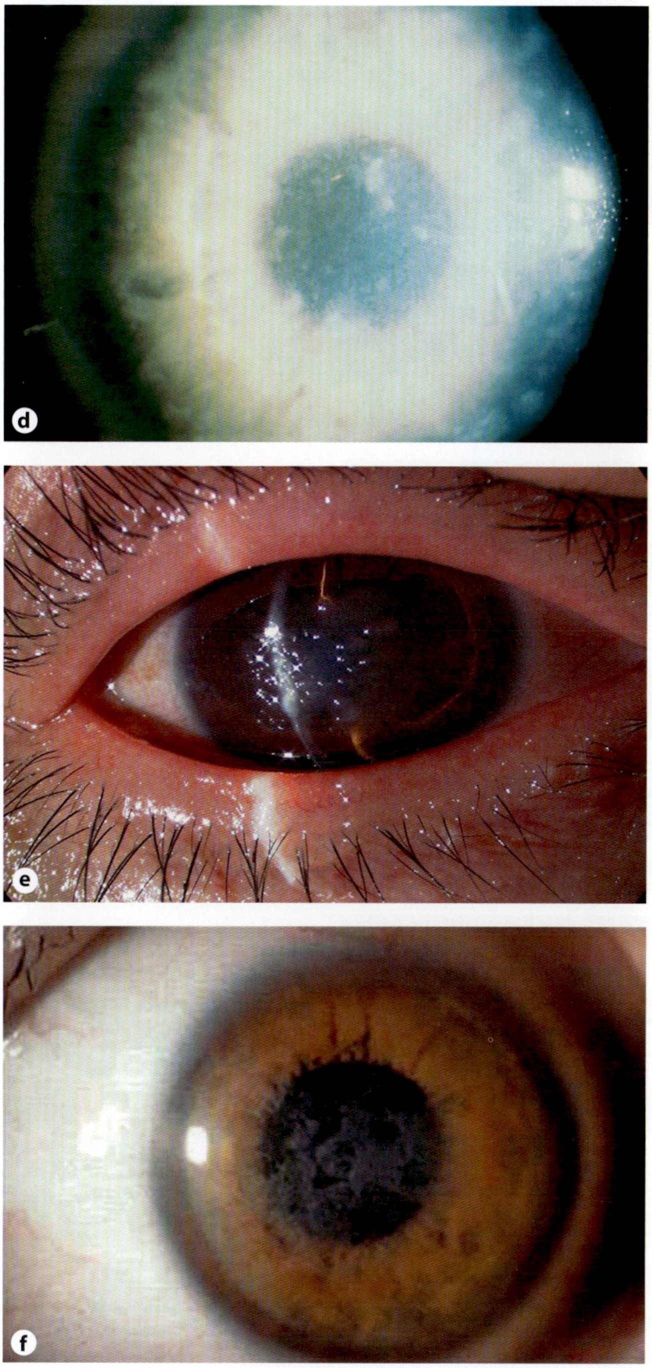

Fig. 5. **d** Multiple flecks and diffuse stromal opacity of macular corneal dystrophy in direct illumination. **e** Mulberry-like opacity of gelatinous drop-like corneal dystrophy in direct illumination. **f** Geographic-like opacity of Reis-Bücklers corneal dystrophy in direct illumination.

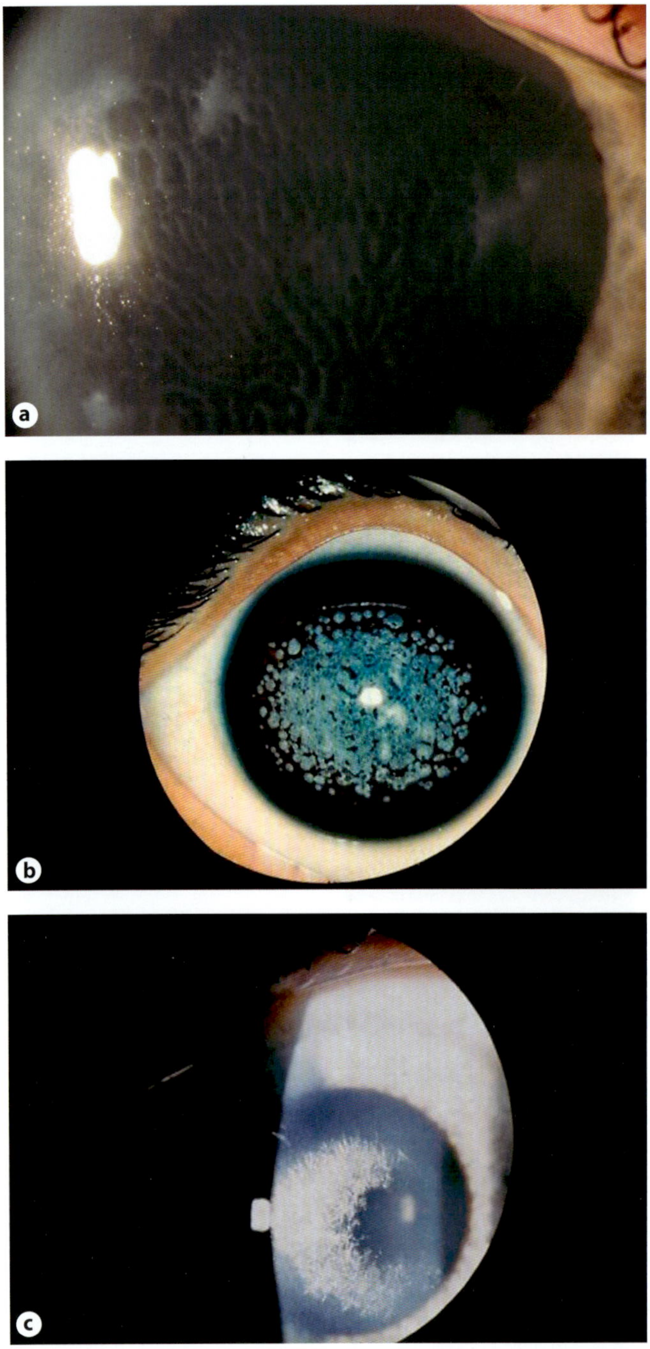

Fig. 6. a Honeycomb-like opacity of Thiel-Behnke corneal dystrophy in direct illumination (courtesy of J.M. Rohrbach). **b** Subepithelial, dense reticular opacity of homozygous GCD2 in direct illumination (courtesy of H.U. Moeller). **c** Central, subepithelial ring consisting of crowded, needle-shaped crystals of Schnyder corneal dystrophy in direct illumination.

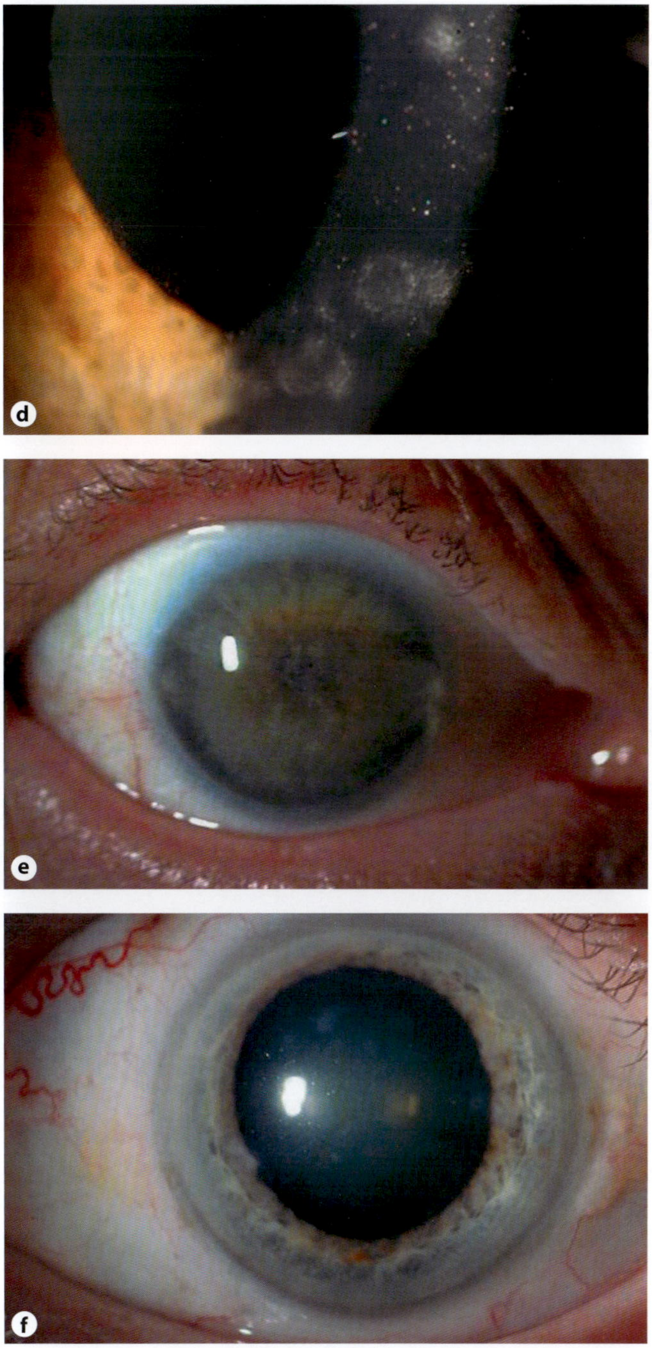

Fig. 6. **d** Monoclonal gammopathy of undetermined significance: solitary, punctiform and multicolored crystals and patch-like opacity in direct illumination. **e** Secondary, subepithelial band keratopathy of XECD in direct illumination. **f** Central, subepithelial diffuse irregular disk of Franceschetti corneal dystrophy in direct illumination

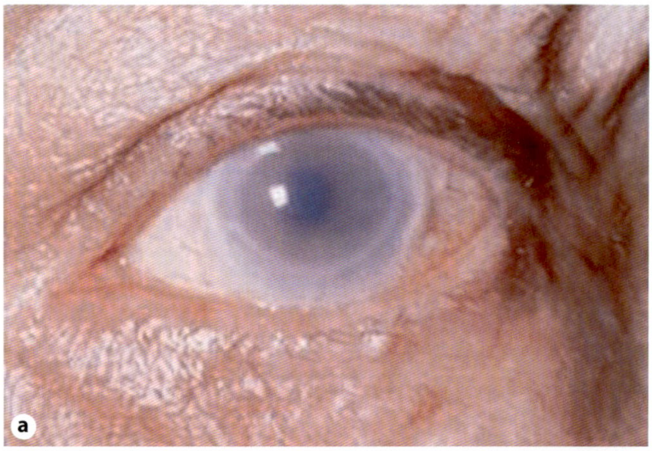

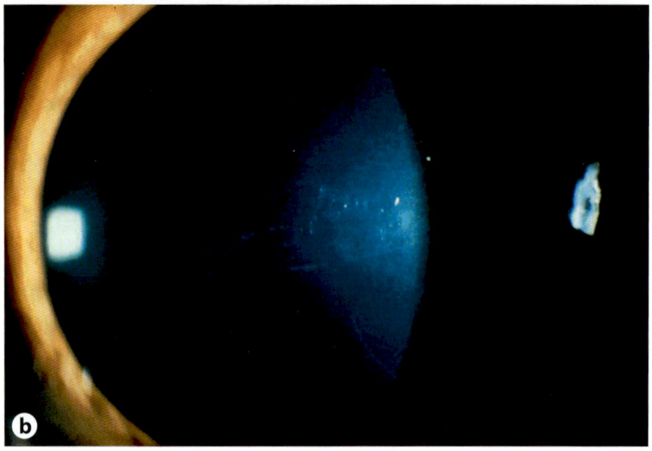

Fig. 7. **a** Lecithin-cholesterol acyltransferase deficiency: moderate diffuse haze and peripheral ring (no true arcus lipoides) in direct illumination. **b** Posterior 'railroad tracks' of PPCD in direct illumination.

Superficial Diffuse Opacities

a Diffuse, central disk or patch-like opacity of Franceschetti corneal dystrophy: directly and indirectly – subepithelial central haze or patch-like opacities (fig. 6f) [14].

b Diffuse, central disk or ring of Schnyder corneal dystrophy [11]: directly and indirectly – subepithelial, central (noncrystalline) milky haze; often associated with arcus lipoides (fig. 2).

c Complete diffuse superficial haze and peripheral ring in lecithin-cholesterol acyltransferase deficiency and fish eye disease (fig. 7a) [15]: directly and indirectly – moderate milky haze and peripheral ring that is not a true arcus lipoides.

d Complete diffuse superficial opacification of mucopolysaccharidoses: directly and indirectly – moderate diffuse haze. Severe extraocular abnormalities.

e Epithelial edema, epithelial bullae and stromal edema in Fuchs endothelial corneal dystrophy: directly and indirectly – epithelial cyst-like changes due to endothelial decompensation (cornea guttata).

Congenital Diffuse Corneal Haze

a Complete stromal haze in CHED types 1 and 2 (CHED2 – autosomal recessive; CHED1 – autosomal dominant): directly and indirectly – severe, ground-glass, milky appearance of the cornea; in CHED1, corneal haze not always congenital but often in the first years; in CHED1, also so-called asymptomatic cases with endothelial moon-crater-like changes and the possibility of late corneal decompensation; thickening of the cornea; usually no increased corneal diameter.

b Complete stromal haze in PPCD (autosomal dominant): directly and indirectly – ground-glass, milky appearance of the cornea; very rare; in about 15% of cases secondary glaucoma; so-called asymptomatic cases with endothelial band-like alterations and the possibility of late corneal decompensation.

c Complete stromal haze in XECD [13]: only in male patients; directly and indirectly – ground-glass, milky haze of the cornea; all affected patients without corneal haze disclose moon-crater-like endothelial changes including male patients with secondary band keratopathy.

d Congenital glaucoma: directly and indirectly – diffuse corneal haziness with enlargement of the eye and occurrence of Descemet's membrane breaks (Haab's striae); increased corneal diameter.

Posterior Band-Like Opacities

a Posterior 'railroad tracks' in PPCD (fig. 7b): directly and indirectly – isolated or multiple posterior bands that can include blister-like lesions combined with varying gray tissue at the level of Descemet's membrane.

Specific Endothelial Alterations

b Posterior dendritic, boomerang-like, circular, comma-like, linear, filiform (cornea farinata), and crystalline-like opacities of pre-Descemet corneal dystrophy [16, 17]: directly and indirectly – very moderate posterior haze.

c Cornea guttata as the compensated stage of Fuchs endothelial corneal dystrophy (fig. 8a): directly and indirectly – regular, multiple drop-like excrescences of Descemet's membrane (beaten metal), often combined with fine endothelial pigmentations or with patches of pigmentation.

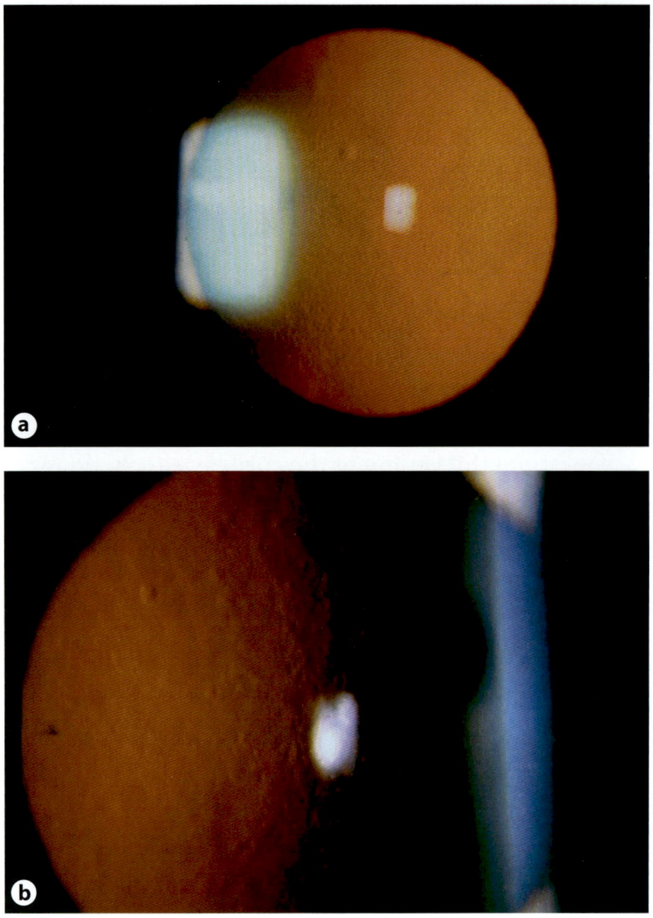

Fig. 8. **a** Cornea guttata in form of regular, multiple drop-like excrescences of Descemet's membrane as the compensated form of Fuchs endothelial corneal dystrophy in indirect illumination. **b** Moon-crater-like, irregular endothelial changes of XECD in indirect illumination.

d Moon-crater-like endothelial changes in CHED1, PPCD, and XECD (male and female patients) (fig. 8b) [13]: directly, but above all indirectly – irregular (in contrast to the regular cornea guttata!), tiny endothelial alterations resembling moon craters.

The presented list of different opacity patterns and units in CDs is supposed to be a bridge for the ophthalmologists to precisely define the corneal opacities of a presumed CD [1]. This bridge makes it easier for them to study the IC3D classification of the CDs [3] and to get more information including adequate differential diagnosis.

References

1 Lisch W, Seitz B: Neue internationale Klassifikation der Hornhautdystrophien und klinische 'Schlüsselbefunde'. Klin Monatsbl Augenheilkd 2008;225:616–622.

2 Wiggs JL: Genotypes need phenotypes. Arch Ophthalmol 2010;128:934–935.

3 Weiss JS, Moeller HU, Lisch W, et al: The IC3D classification of the corneal dystrophies. Cornea 2008; 27(suppl 2):S1–S83.
4 Butros S, Lang GK, Alvarez de Toledo J, et al: Die verschiedenen Trübungsmuster der Lisch-Hornhautdystrophie. Klin Monatsbl Augenheilkd 2006; 223:837–840.
5 Laibson PR: Microcystic corneal dystrophy. Trans Am Ophthalmol Soc 1976;74:488–531.
6 Rosenberg ME, Tervo TM, Gallar J, et al: Corneal morphology and sensitivity in lattice dystrophy type II (familial amyloidosis, Finnish type). Invest Ophthalmol Vis Sci 2001;41:634–641.
7 Weidle EG: Granular corneal dystrophy: two variants; in Ferraz de Olivera LN (ed): Ophthalmology Today. Amsterdam, Elsevier, 1988, pp 617–619.
8 Weidle EG: Klinische und feingewebliche Abgrenzung der Reis-Bücklers'schen Hornhautdystrophie. Klin Monatsbl Augenheilkd 1989;194: 217–226.
9 Weidle EG: Die wabenförmige Hornhautdystrophie (Thiel-Behnke). Neubewertung und Abgrenzung gegenüber der Reis-Bücklersschen Hornhautdystrophie. Klin Monatsbl Augenheilkd 1999;214: 125–135.
10 Moon JW, Kim SW, Kim T, et al: Homozygous granular corneal dystrophy type II (Avellino corneal dystrophy): natural history and progression after treatment. Cornea 2007;26:1095–1100.
11 Weiss JS: Visual morbidity in thirty-four families with Schnyder's corneal dystrophy. Trans Am Soc Ophthalmol 2007;105:1–33.
12 Lisch W, Saikia P, Pitz S, et al: Chameleon-like appearance of immunotactoid keratopathy. Cornea, in press.
13 Schmid E, Lisch W, Philipp W, et al: A new, X-linked endothelial corneal dystrophy. Am J Ophthalmol 2006;141:478–487.
14 Lisch W, Munier F, Schorderet DF, et al: Franceschetti corneal dystrophy (FRCD). Am J Ophthalmol, in press.
15 Weidle EG, Lisch W: Recognizing lecithin cholesterol acyltransferase (LCAT) deficiency at the slitlamp. Arch Ophthalmol 1988;106:1164.
16 Grayson M, Wilbrandt M: Pre-descemet dystrophy. Am J Ophthalmol 1967;64:276–282.
17 Fernandez-Sasso D, Acosta JE, Malbran E: Punctiform and polychromatic pre-Descemet's dominant corneal dystrophy. Br J Ophthalmol 1979; 63:336–338.

Prof. Dr. med. Walter Lisch
Department of Ophthalmology
City Hospital of Hanau
Leimenstrasse 20, DE–63450 Hanau (Germany)
Tel. +49 6181 20649, E-Mail Lisch.Hanau@t-online.de

Lisch W, Seitz B (eds): Corneal Dystrophies.
Dev Ophthalmol. Basel, Karger, 2011, vol 48, pp 24–50

Histological Landmarks in Corneal Dystrophy: Pathology of Corneal Dystrophies

Geeta K. Vemuganti[a] · Varsha M. Rathi[b] · Somasheila I. Murthy[b]

[a]School of Medical Sciences, University of Hyderabad, [b]Cornea and Anterior Segment Service, L.V. Prasad Eye Institute, Hyderabad, India

Abstract

Corneal dystrophies are bilateral, progressive, genetically determined noninflammatory diseases restricted to the cornea. These are characterized by deposition of nonnative protein or other material, both intracellular and extracellular, within the corneal layers. Dystrophies are classified based on the anatomical location of the lesions as: anterior corneal dystrophies (affecting the epithelium and extending into the superficial stroma), stromal dystrophies (which involve the stroma only) and posterior corneal dystrophies (which include the Descemet's membrane and endothelium). Recent additions in the field of genetics and molecular basis of the dystrophies have led to the evolution of a new classification which incorporates genotypic-phenotypic features. While histopathologic study is the gold standard for the diagnosis, various other techniques help provide additional information in this area. Corneal dystrophies can be considered unique as the association of gene-protein disease has been approached both in the forward direction as well as the reverse order. In this chapter, we attempt to highlight the histological features of corneal dystrophies from the cumulative evidence obtained from the study of corneal buttons, enucleated specimens, corneal biopsies, electron microscopic studies, histochemistry and immunohistochemistry.

Corneal dystrophies are a heterogeneous group clinically evident as an opacity or alteration. They are bilateral, progressive, genetically determined noninflammatory diseases restricted to the cornea [1]. Traditionally, dystrophies are classified, based on the anatomical location of the lesions, as anterior corneal dystrophies including the epithelium, basement membrane, Bowman's layer and the superficial stroma, stromal corneal dystrophies which involve the stroma only, and posterior corneal dystrophies which include the Descemet's membrane and endothelium. Recent additions in the field of genetics and molecular basis of the dystrophies have led to the evolution of a new classification which incorporates genotypic-phenotypic features [2].

Weiss et al. [2] in 2008 proposed a classification which is primarily based on the anatomic level of involvement, but additionally each dystrophy has a template summarizing the genetic, clinical and pathologic information (IC3D). Interestingly, it also assigns a number (1–4) which reflects the level of evidence supporting the existence of a given dystrophy.

In this chapter, we refer to the histological, immunohistological and ultrastructural changes observed in various kinds of dystrophies based on the anatomic classification, with an attempt to link it to the recently proposed IC3D classification. Histopathologic studies continue to remain the gold standard in day-to-day practice and as evidenced from the recent classification, they have also influenced the thought process of clinicians and geneticists. Corneal dystrophies can be considered as unique in the sense that the association of gene-protein-disease has been approached both in the forward direction as well as the reverse order.

Although the majority can be diagnosed on clinical examination based on typical clinical features like age of onset, bilaterality, characteristic pattern and depth of opacities, sparing of the limbus and lack of inflammatory signs, nevertheless, the presence of secondary changes like scarring, degeneration and vascularization can mask the clinical features of the dystrophy thus posing diagnostic dilemmas [3, 4]. It is also well known that clinical manifestations vary widely with different phenotypes of the same dystrophy; for example, granular dystrophy has two distinct clinical phenotypes. On the other hand, several infections, inflammatory conditions and scars can show secondary degenerative changes that resemble corneal dystrophies. In this chapter, we attempt to highlight the histological features of corneal dystrophies from the cumulative evidence obtained from the study of corneal buttons, enucleated specimens, corneal biopsies, electron microscopic studies, histochemistry and immunohistochemistry [5–17].

Superficial Corneal Dystrophies: Epithelial and Subepithelial Dystrophies

This group of corneal dystrophies comprises epithelial basement membrane dystrophy (EBMD) which includes maps, fingerprints, dots (earlier known as 'Cogan's dystrophy') and Bron's blebs, Meesmann corneal dystrophy, Lisch epithelial corneal dystrophy, and gelatinous drop-like corneal dystrophy (GDLD). Bowman's layer dystrophies include Reis-Bücklers corneal dystrophy (RBCD), Thiel-Behnke corneal dystrophy (TBCD), and Grayson-Wilbrandt dystrophy as a variant of TBCD. Most of the epithelial dystrophies are diagnosed clinically by slit lamp biomicroscopy or using newer modalities like confocal microscopy [18] and seldom require a biopsy. The source of specimens could be from an occasional therapeutic keratectomy.

Epithelial Basement Membrane Dystrophy

Epithelial basement membrane dystrophy is the most common corneal dystrophy. Incompleteness of the epithelial basement membrane complex is a common fault in most of the anterior corneal dystrophies [19]. It is also known as map-dot-fingerprint-bleb disease. Guerry [20] clinically described fingerprint lines in addition to the classic dot changes in the epithelium described by Cogan et al. [21]. There are other studies wherein EBMD is described as an accumulation of subepithelial material like basement membrane, and horizontally oriented moderately basophilic amorphous material found in the epithelium and under the aberrant basement membrane [22]. Regarding bleb patterns, the material described is fibrinogranular, periodic acid-Schiff (PAS)-positive and a polysaccharide-protein complex as it resists digestion with diastase. The epithelial basement membrane is normal. Sometimes EBMD may be associated with lattice-like lines because of recurrent corneal erosions misleading the diagnosis of lattice dystrophy [23].

The so-called Cogan's dots of EBMD do not have a genetic predisposition and were first described by Cogan as bilateral symmetrical cystic intraepithelial lesions of less than 0.5 mm in diameter. The opacities appeared spontaneously and changed their position. Patients were usually asymptomatic except for intermittent episodes of foreign body sensation [24]. Rodrigues et al. [25] described the pathology of these changes in 1974. The authors found sheet-like aberrant areas of basement membrane extending superficially into the substance of the epithelium. It was also noted that the dots or cysts were composed of intraepithelial lacunae containing cellular debris and pyknotic nucleus. These cells migrated towards the surface and resulted in epithelial erosions. The content of the cysts was PAS-positive material. Also, the basement membrane extended into the epithelium [25]. Guerry [26] reported map-like lesions which did not disappear and reappear due to the deposition of anomalous basement membrane-like material and he concluded that this was part of the same entity. In 1978, Dark [12] concluded, investigating biopsy specimens of 3 corneas, that EBMD, including maps, fingerprints, dots or microcysts and blebs, and Meesmann corneal dystrophy are separate entities.

Imaging Studies. Recently, confocal microscopy has been utilized in the diagnosis of the cystic lesions, and cysts were noted in 9 out of 13 patients. Hernandez-Quintela et al. [18] concluded that confocal microscopy is suitable in identifying cystic lesions but not as sensitive as biomicroscopy.

The bleb type of EBMD was described by Dark [13] in 1977 and is characterized by deposition of a neutral mucopolysaccharide-protein complex as a continuous layer between the basement membrane and Bowman's layer. Clinically, contact lens-induced microcysts show reverse illumination on a slit lamp [27] and may mimic this entity. Light microscopy of the cornea showed a homogenous appearance of the blebs, with a fine granular ultrastructure noted on electron microscopy, suggestive of a friable basement membrane. However, the hemidesmosome system appeared to be normal. Fissures in the bleb material were also noted [13]. Confocal microscopy revealed highly reflective tissue within the intermediate and basal epithelial cell layers corresponding to the abnormal basement membrane extending into the epithelium. There were thin, parallel hyperreflective lines and high-contrast round lesions of various sizes within the epithelium, with distorted basal epithelial cells ranging between 10 and 250 μm within the epithelium, around the abnormal basement membrane. The blebs appeared as circular or oval hyporeflective areas between 40 and 100 μm, at the level of the basal epithelium and Bowman's layer, accompanied by hyperreflective linear structures extending into the epithelium [28].

Meesmann Corneal Dystrophy

Light Microscopy. Meesmann corneal dystrophy is characterized by intraepithelial cysts which are filled with PAS-positive degenerative material that shows autofluorescence in ultraviolet light and stains with the Hale colloidal iron technique for negatively charged substances such as glycosaminoglycans. It is also resistant to diastase and neuraminidase. The irregularity is limited to the corneal epithelium which shows increased thickness, loss of normal architecture, loss of cell polarity, increased amounts of intracellular glycogen, presence of intraepithelial microcysts containing degenerated cells, and in some cases vacuolated epithelial cells [29].

Transmission Electron Microscopy. Transmission electron microscopy (TEM) shows focal aggregations of electron-dense fibrillogranular keratin within the cytoplasm of the corneal epithelium designated as peculiar substance which is surrounded by cytoplasmic filaments and vacuoles [1].

Imaging Studies. Confocal microscopy of the cystic lesions shows hyporeflective round, oval or teardrop areas in the basal epithelial cell layer. The peculiar substance, i.e. fibrillogranular material and tonofilament bundles, appear as reflective spots. The subbasal nerve plexus appears fragmented [30].

Lisch Epithelial Corneal Dystrophy

The epithelial cells in parts of the cornea that correspond to the clinically evident whorl-like opacity have a diffuse cytoplasmic vacuolization. By TEM, the vacuoles are mainly empty but also contain electron-dense whorled inclusions. Scattered areas of vacuolization are seen within the entire epithelium [31, 32]. The clinical appearance of 'cysts' is probably due to clusters of epithelial cells with vacuolar cytoplasmic rarefaction and reduced tonofilaments.

GDLD is one of the most remarkable dystrophies with a striking clinical picture, classical histological appearance and with almost 100% predictability of recurrence. Histologically, it has been classified into 3 forms – mild, moderate and severe. The mild form is characterized by subepithelial amyloid nodules; the moderate form shows amyloid deposits in a sheet-like pattern in the subepithelial region and superficial stroma (fig. 1a). These deposits correspond to the gelatinous masses seen clinically and stain brick red with Congo red stain (fig. 1b). It is interesting to note that despite significant amounts of amyloid being deposited in the anterior stroma and in the subepithelial region, there is no overall increase in the thickness of the cornea. This makes one speculate if there is any specific signaling between the epithelial cells and stromal cells that controls the cumulative corneal thickness. Secondary changes like chronic inflammatory cells, giant cell reaction, scarring and vascularization have frequently been observed [33]. In such situations, it would be difficult to differentiate primary GDLD from secondary deposits of amyloid seen in long-standing cases of corneal edema, scarring or even other dystrophies (fig. 1c) [34].

In addition, fusiform deposits similar to those in lattice corneal dystrophy (LCD) may also form in the deeper stroma [35]. The amyloid contains lactoferrin, but the disease is not linked to the lactoferrin gene. Basement membrane is abnormally thickened and has a band-like appearance [36]. The surrounding stroma shows a large number of thick filamentous proteoglycan deposits [37].

Immunofluorescence Analysis. Tight junction areas of surface cells lacked expression of ZP-1 and occludin and epithelial cells lacked expression of claudin-1 or desmoplakin (desmosome component). Basement membrane-related proteins were widely expressed throughout the basement membrane. Lactoferrin is also expressed in amyloid deposits and the thickened basement membrane [38]. A small amount of keratoepithelin in superficial stroma causes damage of the Bowman's layer and thinning of the epithelium [36]. All these findings indicate that there is a cell-to-cell disturbance as well as a cell-to-substrate disturbance and altered, i.e. increased, superficial epithelial cell membrane permeability [36, 38, 39]. The gelatinous drop-like opacities may sometimes present as band-like rather than drop-like opacities [40, 41].

Immunohistochemical studies revealed a higher staining affinity of subepithelial amyloid for antiapolipoprotein J than for antiapolipoprotien E [42]. Immunohistochemical staining is mildly positive for amyloid AL (light chain), but negative for amyloid AA, AF, AB, and keratin. Thus, the precursor protein of the amyloid deposits in GDLD might derive from immunoglobulins, for example, from the tear film [43]. Spheroidal degeneration which may accompany the amyloid deposits can be distinguished by the absence of immunostaining [38, 44]. It is also suggested that the corneal epithelial cells with GDLD may produce a precursor of amyloid related to protein AA-3 [45, 46].

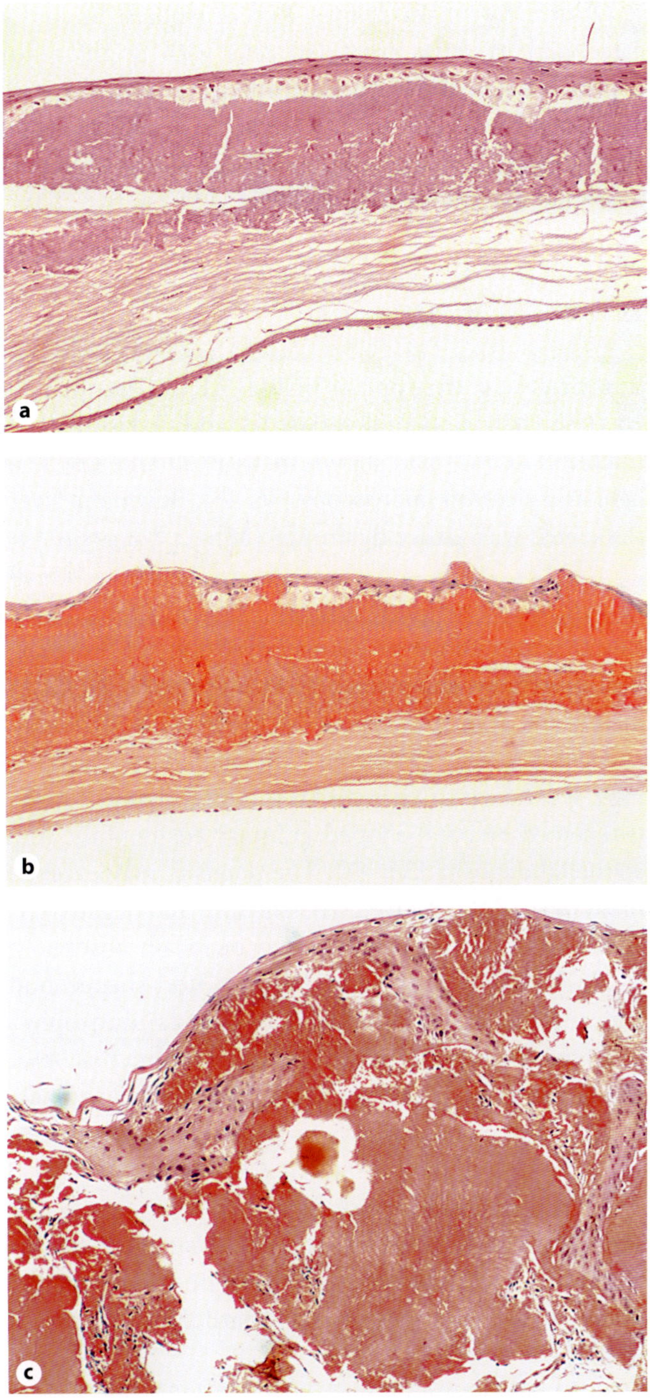

Fig. 1. a Amyloid deposits in a sheet-like pattern extending up to the midstroma in case of GDLD. Hematoxylin and eosin stain. **b** The deposits stain brick red with Congo red stain. **c** A long-standing case of congenital hereditary endothelial corneal dystrophy with secondary amyloid can mimic GDLD.

Other Imaging Modalities. Recent studies on confocal microscopy showed elongated and irregular epithelial cells with bright reflective amyloid material either within or below the epithelium and in the anterior stroma [35].

Recurrence. Recurrence of GDLD in addition to typical features shows abnormally large sulfated proteoglycan and long-spacing collagen with duplication of epithelial basement membrane seen on TEM [42].

Bowman's Layer Dystrophies

Bowman's layer dystrophies include RBCD, granular corneal dystrophy (GCD) type 3 C1, TBCD C1, potential variant C2 and Grayson-Wilbrandt corneal dystrophy C4.2. Küchle et al. [47] had shown that RBCD and TBCD are 2 distinct entities based on light and electron microscopy [36, 47]. Bowman's layer dystrophy may sometimes be associated with lattice dystrophy [48].

Reis-Bücklers Corneal Dystrophy

RBCD is also known as corneal dystrophy of Bowman's layer type 1, geographic corneal dystrophy, superficial GCD, atypical GCD, GCD type 3, and anterior limiting membrane dystrophy type 1 (MIM No. 608470).

Light Electron Microscopy. The epithelium shows edema, degeneration and thinning secondary to changes in the underlying Bowman's layer which is absent and is replaced by band-shaped granular eosinophilic Masson's trichrome-positive subepithelial deposits [36, 47]. The deposits may extend into the anterior stroma. The material is PAS negative, MPS and amyloid negative. The basement membrane of the epithelium may be normal or may be focally absent.

Transmission Electron Microscopy. Rod-shaped bodies are noted and may histologically be a superficial variant of granular dystrophy.

Other Imaging Modalities. On confocal microscopy, deposits are present in the epithelial basal layer and show high reflectivity from small granular material without any shadows. Fine deposits may be noted in the anterior stroma [49].

Thiel-Behnke Corneal Dystrophy

TBCD is also known as corneal dystrophy of Bowman's layer type 2, honeycomb corneal dystrophy, anterior limiting membrane dystrophy type 2, curly fibers corneal dystrophy, and Waardenburg-Jonker corneal dystrophy (MIM No. 602082).

Light Microscopy. Light microscopy [47] shows the epithelium of varying thickness with nonspecific degenerative changes, destruction of Bowman's layer, a subepithelial fibrocellular tissue with an undulant configuration and absence of the epithelial basement membrane in many areas. In advanced stages, the anterior stromal collagen and Bowman's layer may be markedly disorganized and replaced by numerous aggregates. Histopathologically, subepithelial fibrous tissue accumulates in a wave-like configuration.

Transmission Electron Microscopy. The presence of 'curly' collagen fibers with a diameter of 9–15 nm is pathognomonic of TBCD [47]. These are interspersed among normal collagen fibrils in the Bowman's zone and the contiguous superficial corneal stroma. Curly fibers are immunopositive for transforming growth factor β-induced protein (keratoepithelin) in TBCD (5q31).

Other Imaging Modalities. Confocal microscopy shows distinct deposits in the epithelial basal layer, which exhibits homogenous reflectivity with round edges accompanying a dark shadow. This is less reflective as compared to RBCD.

Grayson-Wilbrandt Corneal Dystrophy

Light Microscopy. PAS-positive material is noted between Bowman's layer and the epithelium, which stains negative with Alcian blue and Masson's trichrome stain [50, 51]. Kurome et al. [50] believed that Grayson-Wilbrandt corneal dystrophy is a variant of RBCD, but today we know that it is a variant of TBCD.

Stromal Corneal Dystrophies

This group of corneal dystrophies includes macular corneal dystrophy (MCD), GCD type 1, LCD, Schnyder's corneal dystrophy, fleck corneal dystrophy, congenital stromal corneal dystrophy and posterior amorphous corneal dystrophy. These dystrophies also constitute the most common type of corneal specimens received by the pathologists for histopathologic evaluation. With the advent of lamellar surgeries, the type of specimen is now changing from full-thickness penetrating keratoplasty to lamellar tissues wherein we receive only part of the corneal tissue or multiple fragments of shredded tissue making it difficult to evaluate the architectural details.

Granular Corneal Dystrophy Type 1

GCD type 1 is also known as classic GCD and corneal dystrophy Groenouw type 1 (MIM No. 121900).

Light Microscopy. Patchy, crystal-like eosinophilic to orangish deposits in the corneal stroma are hallmarks of GCD (fig. 2a, b). These deposits are predominantly extracellular and stain as brilliant red with Masson's trichrome (fig. 2c). An interesting unpublished observation made by one of the authors (G.K.V.) was that the Masson-stained section of GCD under polarized filters shows bright autofluorescence (fig. 2d, e). In histopathologically confirmed recurrences, the deposits are noted to be superficial to Bowman's layer in subepithelial nonvascularized fibrocollagenous tissue with fibroblasts almost certainly of host origin. The rare characteristic deposits within the

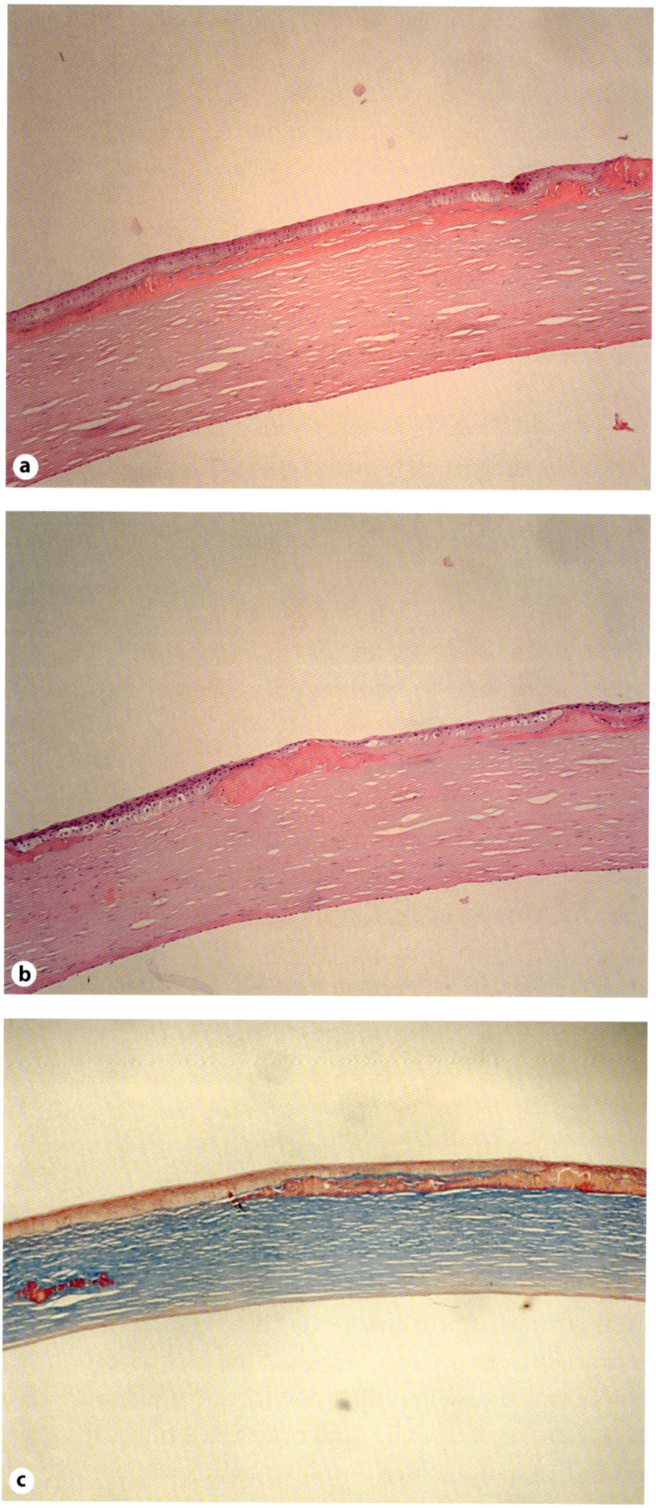

Fig. 2. **a**, **b** Section of the cornea in granular dystrophy shows predominantly subepithelial location of the confluent eosinophilic to orange deposits (**a**) and is also distributed in the deeper stroma (**b**). Hematoxylin and eosin stain. **c** Masson's trichrome stain shows brilliant red deposits located subepithelially and also in the deeper stroma.

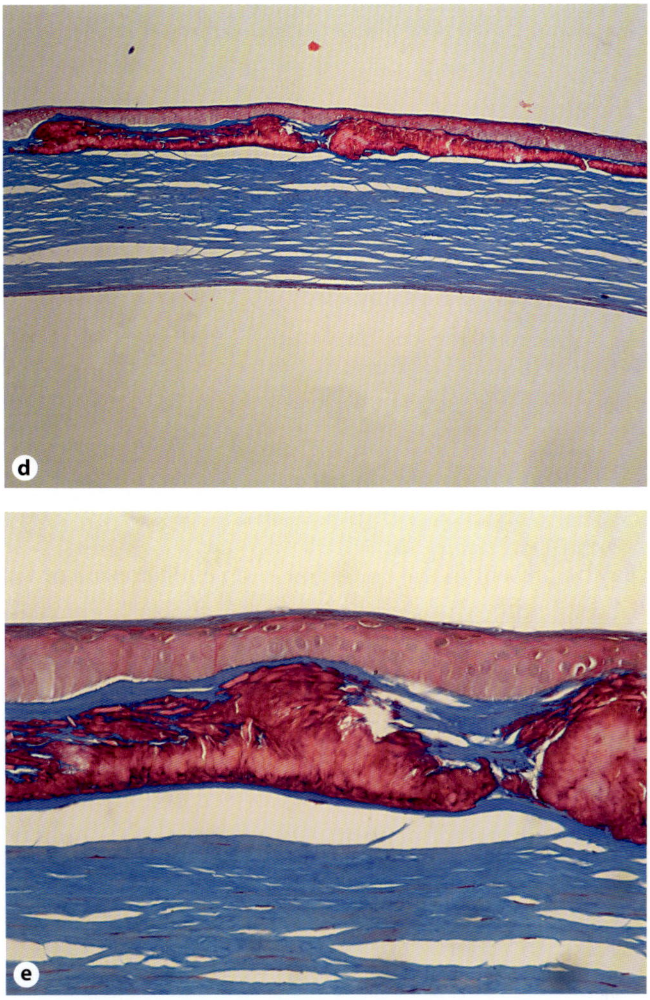

Fig. 2. d, **e** Masson's trichrome-stained section of GCD shows bright autofluorescence under polarizing filters, seen under low (**d**) and high magnification (**e**).

peripheral stroma of the donor cornea probably result from an invasion of the graft by corneal fibroblasts (keratocytes) of the recipient. Fibrous tissue without vascularization is present between the epithelium and Bowman's layer and contains deposits characteristic of granular dystrophy in both light and electron microscopy [52].

Transmission Electron Microscopy. Small intraepithelial cytoplasmic granules are noted to be rimmed by 15-nm particles, while larger deposits were often membrane-bound. The granules were closely associated with tonofilaments and also show ultrastructural similarities to keratohyaline; the granules had central electron-dense, discrete rod-shaped or trapezoid bodies (fig. 3), partially surrounded by 9- to 10-nm tubular microfibrils [53]. Cross-sectional profiles of the corneal deposits are usually irregularly shaped, but sometimes hexagonal measuring 100–500 nm in diameter. Clusters of these elongated bodies occur particularly in the superficial corneal stroma and they

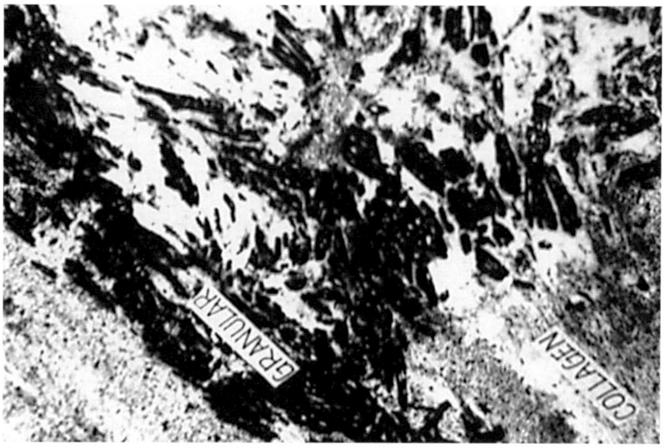

Fig. 3. Electron microscopy in GCD shows central, electron-dense discreet rod-shaped bodies.

may be present in the epithelial intercellular space or within degenerated basal epithelial cells. Some rod-shaped structures appear homogenous without a discernible inner structure; others, however, are composed of an orderly array of closely packed filaments (70–100 nm in width) orientated parallel to their long axis, while others appear moth-eaten with variable-shaped cavities containing fine filaments. Some superficial and most deep stromal deposits do not all possess the rod-shaped configuration. Descemet's membrane and the corneal endothelium are unremarkable, and so is the cornea between the deposits. Disintegrated squamous epithelial cells with extracellular granules were often intermixed with cytoplasmic organelles suggestive of an epithelial origin of the granular dystrophic deposits in recurrent granular dystrophy [54] in addition to the presence of intracellular rod and trapezoidal crystalline granules.

A variant of granular dystrophy, also termed 'Avellino corneal dystrophy' may be associated with the presence of amyloid. The current name for this disorder is granular corneal dystrophy type 2. Recently, oxidative stress has been proven to be responsible for the pathogenesis of GCD type 2. Decreased catalase is responsible for the oxidative damage [55].

Immunohistochemistry. With the Wilder reticulin stain, the accumulations contain tangles of argyrophilic fibers. The deposits react with histochemical methods for protein as well as with antibodies to transforming growth factor β-induced protein. The granules stain positively with luxol fast blue and are reported to stain positively with antibodies to microfibrillar protein. Human intercellular adhesion molecule 1 was expressed focally in epithelial cells and in keratocytes, and expressed diffusely in endothelial cells [56].

Other Imaging Modalities. Confocal microscopy findings near Bowman's layer may be similar in all 3 stromal dystrophies [49]. Spectral optical coherence tomography shows that multiple hyperreflective changes can be seen secondary to amyloid deposits [57].

Recurrence of Dystrophy. Granular structures are deposited in the posterior stroma with partially digested keratocytes and abnormal proteoglycan is present [58].

Macular Corneal Dystrophy

MCD is also known as corneal dystrophy Groenouw type 2, and Fehr corneal dystrophy (MIM No. 217800).

Light Microscopy. The histopathology of MCD is characteristic. Intracytoplasmic accumulations occur within the keratocytes and corneal endothelium, but the corneal epithelium is spared (fig. 4a). The accumulations stain positively with histochemical stains for glycosaminoglycans, such as PAS, Alcian blue (fig. 4b), and metachromatic dyes, and possess an affinity for colloidal iron. The accumulations also stain with the PAS/thiocarbohydrazide/silver proteinate and the periodic acid-methenamine silver techniques. Histopathologically, MCD is typified by an intracellular storage of glycosaminoglycans within keratocytes and the corneal endothelium combined with an extracellular deposition of similar material in the corneal stroma and Descemet's membrane (fig. 4c). Guttae are common on Descemet's membrane. Numerous electron-transparent lacunae are randomly distributed throughout MCD corneas. The collagen fibrils have a normal diameter but their packing differs between specimens.

Vital staining with fluorescent dye acridine orange detects abnormalities of lysozymes and the corneal fibroblasts of patients with MCD show the same as control but the mucopolysaccharidosis patients' cells are easily and accurately separated from other fibroblasts [59].

Electron Microscopy. Cuprolinic blue staining for sulfated proteoglycans shows 4.6-A periodic repeats in MCD corneas residing in large sulfated proteoglycan filaments that may contain chondroitin/dermatan sulfate and keratan sulfate or keratan components [42]. Intracytoplasmic vacuoles are a distinct ultrastructural feature of the keratocytes and with appropriate tissue fixation delicate fibrillogranular material can be discerned within the vesicles. Some corneal endothelial cells contain similar material. Numerous electron-lucent lacunae are randomly distributed throughout corneas and some lacunae are filled with clusters of abnormal sulfated chondroitinase ABC nonsusceptible proteoglycan filaments. The collagen fibrils have a normal diameter, but the interfibrillar spacing of collagen fibrils in affected corneas is less than that in the normal cornea. This close packing of collagen fibrils seems to be responsible for the reduced corneal thickness in MCD. The anterior banded portion of Descemet's membrane which forms in utero is of normal thickness and has an unremarkable ultrastructure, whereas the posterior layer usually contains numerous corneal guttae. Another interesting aspect of MCD is the involvement of the endothelial cells by the deposits (fig. 4c) that is believed to be a secondary involvement, which is of clinical relevance in view of the increasing use of lamellar keratoplasty by some surgeons. In

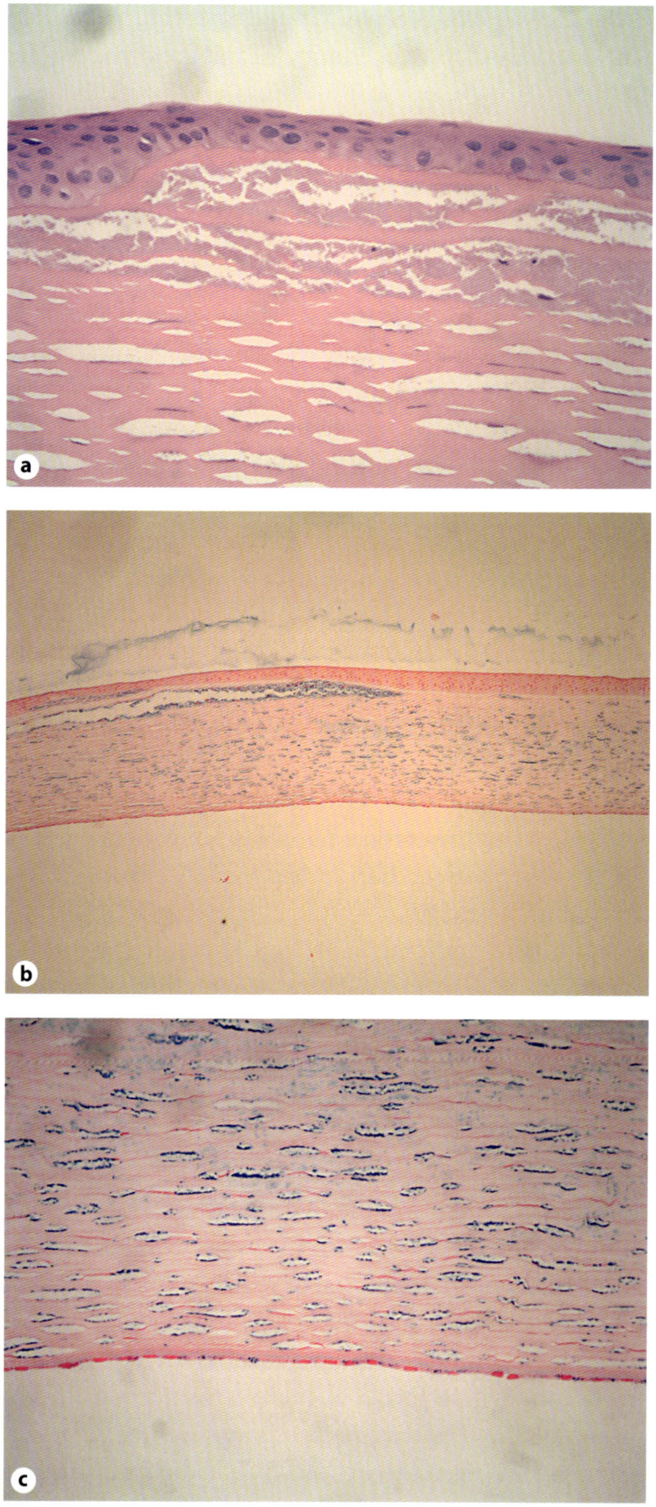

Fig. 4. **a** MCD under hematoxylin and eosin stain shows granular deposits accumulated below the epithelial basement membrane and also in keratocytes. **b**, **c** Alcian blue stain shows that the deposits are noted throughout the stroma (**b**) and also in the cytoplasm of the endothelial cells (**c**).

a retrospective study conducted at our institute [unpubl. data], we analyzed the visual outcomes and complication rates of deep anterior lamellar keratoplasty in MCD. In our series, 21 eyes of 20 patients were followed up at 1 year. Seventy percent achieved visual acuity of 20/40 or better and 80% of the grafts remained clear. Only 1 graft failed due to endothelial decompensation. Our data suggest that the presence of these deposits in the endothelial cells may not necessarily compromise the endothelial function.

Immunohistochemistry. MCD can be classified into 3 different immunophenotypes according to the presence and distribution of sulfated keratan sulfate in the cornea and serum levels of sulfated keratan sulfate [60]. MCD type 1 has no detectable keratan sulfate in the serum or cornea, MCD type 2 has normal amounts of keratan sulfate in the serum and cornea, whereas the third type (MCD type 1A) lacks detectable antigenic keratan sulfate in the serum, but has stainable keratan sulfate in the keratocytes. In a study conducted by our group, it was found that MCD type 1 was the predominant immunophenotype in the Indian population studied followed by type 1A and then type 2 [61]. A new phenotype of MCD was also identified with low AgKS levels and stromal presence of AgKS protein suggesting more immunophenotypic heterogeneity than identified so far [61, 62]. Based on the work of Sultana et al. [61], it appears that absence of correlation of immunophenotypes and genotypes warrants further exploration to understand the pathobiology of the disease.

Keratocyte apoptosis as measured by the number of apoptotic keratocytes using the TUNEL assay method showed that it may be a concomitant or pathogenic factor only in MCD, but the triggering pathway for the apoptosis is unknown [56]. Subgroups of MCD can be identified based on the immunoreactivity to keratan sulfate antibodies [63].

Monoclonal antibody against keratan sulfate was used for immunofluorescent staining. The anti-keratan sulfate monoclonal antibody did not stain the corneas with primary MCD and staining was very weak in recurrence of MCD indicating absence of sulfated keratin.

Transmission Electron Microscopy. TEM reveals 2 types of vacuoles which contain either fibrillar or amorphous material. The vacuoles may be flattened. Cytoplasmic organelles of the cells are normal as well as the junctions [63, 64]. On electron microscopy, the endothelial cells in MCD are thin and contain empty vacuoles and numerous granules that stain with Alcian blue and periodic acid fuchsin [63]. The electron-lucent areas presumably contain extracellular deposits of glycosaminoglycans which dissolve during tissue processing. The stroma of MCD corneas contains congregations of cuprolinic blue-stained filaments which vary both in size and in electron density. Increased electron-dense small areas of small-sized basal epithelial cells with few organelles in the overlying epithelium have also been noted, especially in patients who have increased photophobia clinically [65].

Lattice Corneal Dystrophy Type 1

LCD type 1 is also known as Biber-Haab-Dimmer dystrophy (MIM No. 122000).

Light Microscopy. Lattice linear and branching structures about 40–80 μm in width with changing reflectivity and poorly demarcated margins are visible in the stroma and are typical of LCD [56]. Amyloid deposits occur throughout the corneal stroma and appear as fusiform deposits (fig. 5a) that coincide with the lattice pattern of lines and other opacities noted clinically [25]. Long-standing cases can also show secondary changes like spheroidal degeneration (fig. 5b), scarring and vascularization. Like in GDLD, these deposits are congophilic and show apple green birefringence and dichroism when viewed under 2 polarizing filters.

Electron Microscopy. The deposits stain positively with antibodies to protein AP and negatively with antibodies to kappa and lambda immunoglobulin light chains.

Immunohistochemistry. Only the epithelial cells and endothelium are intensively positive for intercellular adhesion molecule 1 [56]. E-selectin was not present on any layer of the corneal specimens. E-cadherin was observed only in the epithelium of all 3 types of corneal dystrophies. The authors concluded that adhesion molecules may be involved in the pathogenesis of corneal stromal dystrophies [56].

Granular Corneal Dystrophy Type 2

GCD type 2 is also known as Avellino corneal dystrophy, and combined granular-lattice corneal dystrophy (MIM No. 607541).

The presence of both hyaline and amyloid deposits resulted in the diagnosis of combined GCD and LCD [66]. These deposits show positivity to Masson's trichrome stain, negative staining or faint staining with Congo red, but no birefringence under polarized light, or fluorescence with thioflavin T as was reported in a case of recurrence after laser-assisted in situ keratomileusis (LASIK) [67]. The deposits in this combination dystrophy appear to be much bigger than the deposits seen in LCD type 1 [68].

Recurrence of GCD Type 2. Corneal stromal deposits in the LASIK flaps displayed bright red color staining with Masson's trichrome and negative staining with Congo red, which suggests that hyaline is the main component localizing to the transforming growth factor β-induced protein deposits rather than amyloid in GCD type 2.

Central Cloudy Dystrophy of François (MIM No. 217600)

Light microscopy shows staining for acid mucopolysaccharidosis [69]. Material within the vacuoles shows intense reactivity with Alcian blue and colloidal iron stains, consistent with glycosaminoglycan deposition.

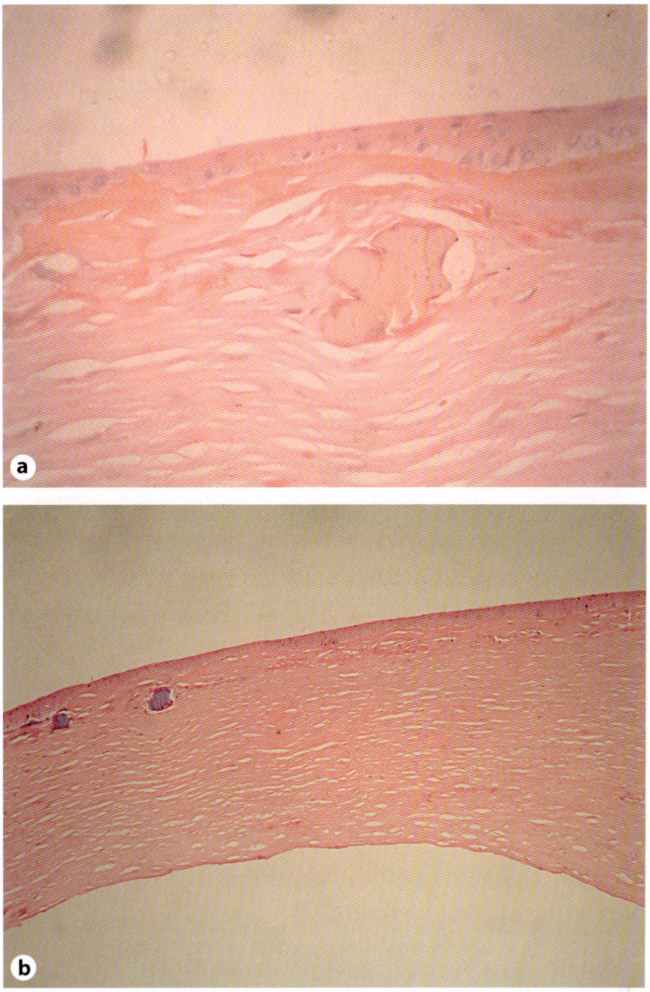

Fig. 5. **a** Hematoxylin and eosin stain in LCD shows fusiform deposits within the corneal stroma. **b** Amphophilic deposits suggestive of spheroidal degeneration are also noted in the anterior stroma, in a specimen from long-standing LCD.

Transmission Electron Microscopy. Extracellular vacuoles with fibrillogranular material and electron-dense deposits are found in and around keratocytes suggestive of amyloid [69].

Fleck Corneal Dystrophy (François-Neetens Speckled Corneal Dystrophy, MIM No. 121850)

Corneal tissue with fleck corneal dystrophy has rarely been examined, but some keratocytes contain fibrillogranular material within intracytoplasmic vacuoles or pleomorphic electron-dense and membranous intracytoplasmic inclusions. The stored material reacts positively with Alcian blue, colloidal iron, Sudan black B and oil red

O stains and is partially sensitive to hyaluronidase and β-galactosidase. It has the histochemical attributes of glycosaminoglycans and lipids. Extracellular alterations are rare, but foci of wide-spaced collagen have been observed [70].

Transmission Electron Microscopy. TEM shows single membrane-limited inclusions containing fine granular material in the affected cells. Some keratocytes contain pleomorphic electron-dense and membranous intracytoplasmic inclusions.

Confocal Microscopy. Confocal microscopy shows refractile bodies with swollen keratocytes and normal stroma [71] and intracellular deposits throughout the stroma in fleck dystrophy [72].

Schnyder's Corneal Dystrophy

Schnyder's corneal dystrophy is also known as Schnyder's crystalline corneal dystrophy, crystalline stromal dystrophy, Schnyder's crystalline dystrophy sine crystals, and hereditary crystalline stromal dystrophy of Schnyder (MIM No. 21800).

Light Microscopy. Birefringent cholesterol crystals and associated neutral fats accumulate within keratocytes and extracellularly, corresponding to the crystals observed clinically. The lipid is also present in Bowman's layer, between the superficial corneal lamellae and dispersed within the stroma among the collagen fibrils. The lipid deposits in Schnyder's corneal dystrophy comprise mainly multilamellar vesicles containing unesterified cholesterol and phospholipids, with a lesser contribution of cholesteryl ester lipid droplets [73, 74]. The lipid deposits within the cornea are predominantly phospholipids and cholesterol (esterified and unesterified). The predominant phospholipid is sphingomyelin [75].

Electron Microscopy. Numerous ovoid electron-lucent areas suggestive of lipid and focal endothelial cell discontinuities are noted [73, 74, 76].

Confocal Microscopy. Large bright reflective crystalline material is seen between the anterior to midstroma [77].

Posterior Corneal Dystrophies (Endothelial Dystrophies)

These include Fuchs endothelial corneal dystrophy (FECD), posterior polymorphous corneal dystrophy (PPCD), congenital hereditary endothelial corneal dystrophy (CHED) and X-linked endothelial corneal dystrophy (XECD).

Endothelial dystrophies are inherited conditions that affect the endothelial cells of the cornea and thereby resulting in corneal edema and thickening of Descemet's membrane. There are 3 main endothelial dystrophies: CHED, FECD and PPCD. The manifestations of loss or dysfunction of the endothelium are in the form of reduced endothelial cell count, pleomorphism in size and shape of endothelial cells, thickening of Descemet's membrane, corneal edema and changes secondary to long-standing edema. The spectrum of these morphologic changes depends on the age of onset, rate of progression, type of inheritance and other local or iatrogenic factors. The specimens obtained in case of endothelial dystrophies include corneal buttons from penetrating keratoplasty, and peeled off Descemet's membrane from endothelial keratoplasty (fig. 6a, b) (like Descemet's stripping endothelial keratoplasty). Clinically, an important tool to evaluate endothelial changes is specular microscopy which helps in the examination of endothelium including pleomorphism, polymegathism and gross guttata changes [78].

Fuchs Endothelial Corneal Dystrophy

FECD is also known as endoepithelial corneal dystrophy (MIM No. 136800). Fuchs' dystrophy corneas had decreased AQP1 [79].

Light Microscopy. In advanced cases, abnormalities are found in all layers of the cornea, but consistent abnormalities involve the corneal endothelium and Descemet's membrane, its basement membrane. The epithelium shows intracellular and basal cell edema, hypertrophy, with breaks in the basement membrane, thickening, irregularity and reduplication and epithelial ingrowth [80]. Bowman's layer may be absent or show discontinuity, with adhesions between the basement membrane and underlying stroma. The subepithelial region may show the presence of a fibrous or fibrovascular pannus in long-standing cases. The stroma shows a decrease in the normal clefts, increased thickness and paler staining due to edema. There may be a decrease in keratocytic nuclei. The underlying abnormality results in a decline in the number of functional endothelial cells, premature corneal endothelial cell degeneration and apoptosis. Melanosomes are often found within the endothelial cells. The corneal endothelium is attenuated over the guttata excrescences and abnormal endothelial cells have widened intercellular spaces, swollen mitochondria, a dilated rough endoplasmic reticulum, and melanosomes. A posterior collagenous layer due to secretion of basement membrane material from the endothelium is seen. This material may project above the surface in the anterior chamber. The endothelial cells are absent or may be thinned out (fig. 6a, b). Multiple excrescences (guttae) of differing size and shape are evident on the posterior surface of Descemet's membrane and protrude into the anterior chamber. Some guttae are mushroom or anvil shaped. Others are multilaminar warts or are buried in the multilaminar extracellular matrix. The guttae are typically more confluent and more centrally located than the guttae of aging, which characteristically involve predominantly the peripheral cornea (Hassall-Henle warts). Fissures within some guttae are penetrated by cellular debris. The distribution of the guttae can be visualized in flat preparations of Descemet's membrane using phase contrast microscopy or scanning electron microscopy. Descemet's membrane is also multilayered and often irregularly thickened (2- to 4-fold) due to an excessive accumulation of collagen especially where the guttae are most abundant. A multilaminar collagenous layer which stains with variable intensity with the PAS stain is commonly

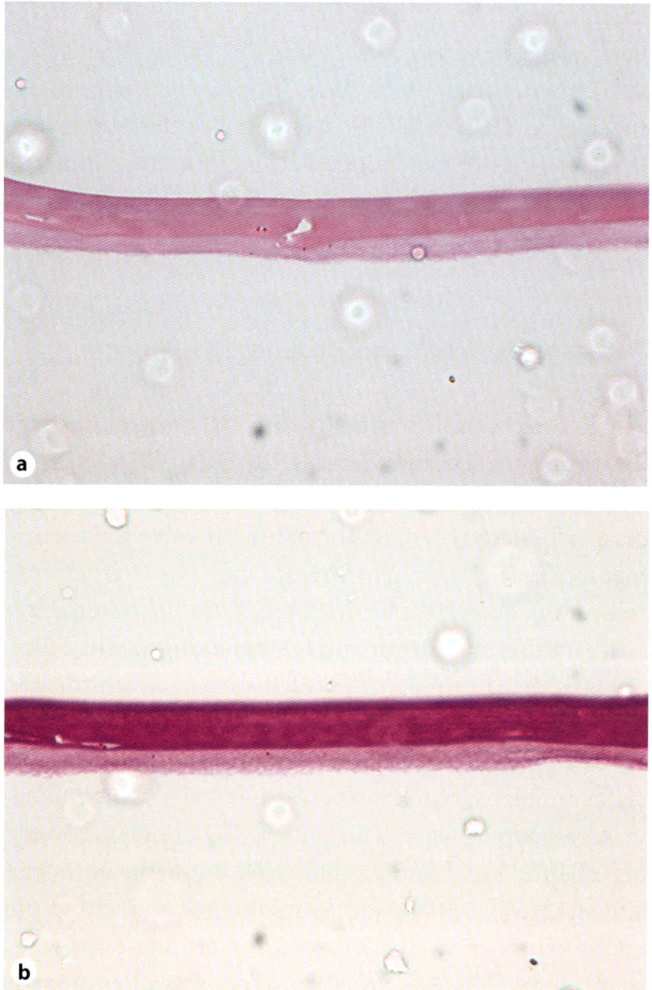

Fig. 6. a, **b** Thickened Descemet's membrane with prominent multilaminar collagenous layer and loss of endothelial cells in FECD (Descemet's stripping endothelial keratoplasty specimen). Seen with hematoxylin and eosin stain (**a**) and PAS stain (**b**).

present. Some subjects with FECD have multilaminar connective tissue posterior to Descemet's membrane, but without corneal guttae.

Transmission Electron Microscopy. Condensed nucleus and decreased cell size suggestive of apoptosis plays an important role in the degeneration of endothelium and the authors concluded that further studies are required to confirm the role of apoptosis in the etiopathogenesis of FECD [81]. Descemet's membrane has a normal 3-μm-thick anterior banded layer and a normal nonbanded portion, but posteriorly it contains fusiform bundles and sheets of wide-spacing (100-nm) collagen with a macroperiodicity of 55 or 100 nm within amorphous material and manifests subbands with a periodicity of about 30–40 nm. Horizontal fibrils run perpendicular to the vertical bands. The wide-spacing collagen forms a hexagonal pattern, which is evident in tangential sections. This pattern is identical to that observed in horizontal sections of the normal anterior banded Descemet's membrane. Tissue specimens in advanced cases contain a layer consisting of loosely packed thin collagen fibrils (20–30 nm in diameter) with a 64-nm banding scattered within basement membrane-like material. Groups of 10- to 20-nm-diameter collagen fibrils are found next to the wide-spacing collagen and may fuse with the horizontal fibrils of the wide-spacing collagen.

Immunohistochemistry. Fibrinogen/fibrin has been noted in the posterior collagenous layer in FECD, but not in normal Descemet's membrane. Tenascin C and fibrillin 1 are expressed in all eyes of bullous keratopathy and in about 50% of eyes with FECD in the fibrocellular extracellular matrix, and basement membrane complex [82], an immunohistochemical study on selected cases of FECD as well as in situ hybridization using labeled sense and antisense *TGFBI* oligonucleotide probes were performed. This study disclosed the presence of transforming growth factor β-induced protein in the subepithelial corneal matrix and in the posterior collagenous layer of FECD.

Decreased immunostaining for NA^+/K^+-ATPase α subunits was seen in almost two thirds of corneas with aphakic or pseudophakic bullous keratopathy and FECD but endothelial staining was normal [82].

Posterior Polymorphous Corneal Dystrophy

PPCD is also known as posterior polymorphous dystrophy, and Schlichting dystrophy (MIM No. 122000).

Light Microscopy. Unlike FECD, corneal guttae are not present on the Descemet's membrane. Sometimes edema of the corneal epithelium and stroma occur, and the anterior cornea may become scarred and develop calcific band keratopathy. Corneal tissue has only been examined in cases of PPCD with glaucoma or those that are severe enough to require a penetrating keratoplasty. The aberrant PPCD endothelium has both simple and squamous stratified epithelium (fig. 7).

Transmission Electron Microscopy. A major morphologic feature of PPCD is the replacement of corneal endothelium with cells having epithelial attributes. Instead of an endothelial monolayer, the posterior cornea is lined by variable numbers of stratified squamous epithelial cells having tonofilaments, cytokeratin and desmosomes. These epithelial cells have numerous microvilli, but unlike normal corneal epithelium, microplicae are not a feature. Descemet's membrane is multilaminar and irregularly thickened and occasionally with focal nodular excrescences, but they differ from the corneal guttae that characterize FECD. Granular deposits in the posterior stroma and a fibrillary zone are noted between the stroma and Descemet's membrane. The Descemet's membrane is thickened with a normal fetal and adult zone and an intermediate zone of long and short collagen fibers and fibrils. Histology showed delamination with 3 layers. Cells towards the anterior chamber were multilayered and had numerous microvilli and were linked with desmosomes suggestive of epithelial cell type. These cells are hypothesized to be of mesenchymatous origin

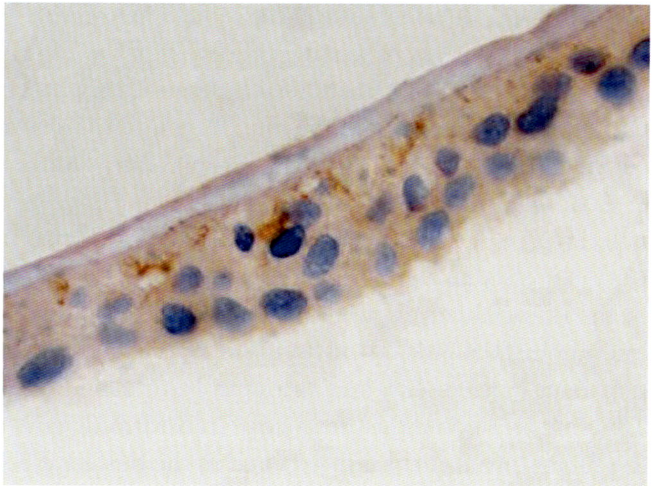

Fig. 7. Light microscopy shows aberrant endothelial cells in a case of PPCD with a stratified layer of cells. Hematoxylin and eosin stain, high magnification.

[83]. In fetal cornea, it was shown that the Descemet's membrane was normal under the normal endothelial cells and it was thinner or absent under the epithelial-like cells [84]. Epithelial-like endothelial cells line the oval or slit-like spaces in the posterior stroma [85]. That the banded anterior layer of Descemet's membrane is present and of normal thickness suggests that the abnormality of the corneal endothelium in PPCD does not become manifest until late in gestation.

Immunohistochemistry. The abnormal endothelial cells show strong immunostaining for a wide variety of cytokeratins (CK3/12, CK4, CK5/6, CK10/13, CK14, CK16 and CK17), but express predominantly cytokeratin 7 and cytokeratin 19 [86].

Other Imaging Modalities. Confocal microscopy shows cracks with polymegathism and pleomorphism in eyes with PPCD and associated guttata [87]. When PPCD recurs, it appears similar in the graft [88]. The bands of PPCD show a thickened Descemet's membrane between the edges and a thinned Descemet's membrane outside as against Haab's striae which appear as a thin area between the thick, curly Descemet's membrane. Also, blebs may be the only associated sign typical of PPCD with band [89].

Congenital Hereditary Endothelial Dystrophy

There is CHED type 1, which is autosomal dominant (MIM No. 121700), and CHED type 2 (autosomal recessive), also known as Maumenee corneal dystrophy (MIM No. 217700).

Light Microscopy. Light microscopy is characterized by thickened Descemet's membrane and normal endothelial cell counts but an abnormal endothelial morphology with irregular and multinucleated cells containing abnormal cell organelles. The entire button is thickened due to edema (fig. 8a). The Descemet's membrane alone is about 16–18 μm thick with deposition of fibrillogranular material on the posterior half [90]. It may be associated with GDLD [91]. The histopathology of CHED type 1 and CHED type 2 is similar, but subtle differences in the thickness of collagen in Descemet's membrane have been described. In CHED type 1, a posterior collagenous layer of fibrillary collagen contributes to the thickness of Descemet's membrane. CHED type 2 cases show an increased tendency for the abnormal endothelium to synthesize a homogenous, posterior, nonbanded Descemet's membrane. The cornea shows increased thickness due to extensive stromal edema with some enlargement of collagen fibrils. These changes, together with the decreased fibril density, scatter light and result in a ground-glass appearance of the cornea. The endothelial cells are scant or degenerated when present (fig. 8b). In an unpublished study by the authors, the thickness of the cornea, the Descemet's membrane thickness and the endothelial cells present on the section were measured in autosomal recessive CHED. The results showed that the mean endothelial cell count was 63 cells in CHED type 2, whereas it was 327 cells in aged matched controls. The Descemet's membrane was nearly 4 times thicker (fig. 8b) when compared to control (fig. 8c) (13.5 vs. 3.5 μm in controls).

Immunohistochemistry. The abnormal endothelium in both PPCD and CHED expresses similar cytokeratins, including cytokeratin 7, which is not present in normal endothelium or surface epithelium suggesting a shared origin for both PPCD and CHED [92].

Dilemmas in Dystrophies

There are several unanswered questions that arise while making a diagnosis of corneal dystrophies. The histopathologic spectrum of dystrophies in all stages is variable, since many of these specimens are removed from patients with advanced stages of the disease. Information on rare cases and many anterior stromal dystrophies is obtained mostly from postmortem material due to limited access to corneal specimens. For example, histologic diagnosis of so-called Avellino dystrophy was made in a patient who underwent LASIK, clinically unsuspected of this condition preoperatively. Postoperatively, the patient manifested the dystrophy, which was limited to the area below the anterior stromal flap. In terms of management of the dystrophy, newer surgical modalities such as lamellar surgeries, like superficial or phototherapeutic keratectomy or lamellar keratoplasty, are now considered as the surgical modality of choice for epithelial and anterior stromal dystrophies. In such instances, the pathologist may or may not receive the dissected lamellae of corneal tissue. Another issue pertaining to lamellar surgeries is the involvement of the residual layers. For example, it is well known that the endothelial cells are involved in MCD, with documented presence of Alcian blue staining within the cytoplasm of endothelial cells. Despite

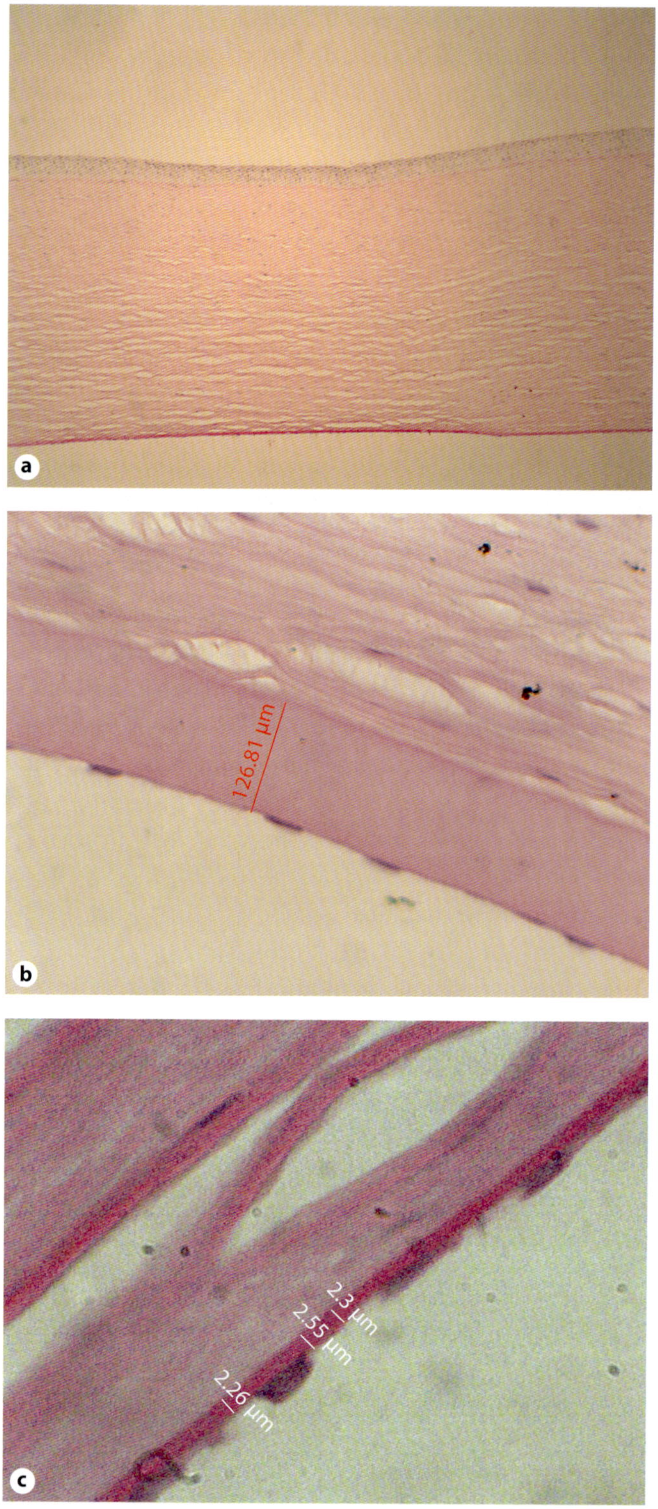

Fig. 8. **a** Light microscopy in a case of CHED under low magnification shows increased thickening due to stromal edema (PAS stain). **b**, **c** Under high magnification, the characteristic thickened Descemet's membrane from a case of autosomal recessive CHED is noted (**b**), with scant endothelial cells, when compared with normal Descemet's membrane (**c**). The thickness of the Descemet's membrane is measured in both specimens.

this, deep anterior lamellar keratoplasty, which has several advantages over penetrating keratoplasty, is performed in MCD, and the early clinical results so far have been encouraging. The long-term survival and function of the residual and affected endothelial cells are not known.

In corneal endothelial dystrophies, endothelial replacements have become the treatment of choice, in the absence of stromal scarring. These procedures are still subject to the risk of rejection and failure. The specimens of a failed endothelial keratoplasty would perhaps provide new and useful information about graft rejection.

The relationship between PPCD and CHED still remains uncertain despite distinct light microscopical, ultrastructural and immunohistochemical differences between these conditions. Inspite of the recognition of patchy epithelial-like alterations of the corneal endothelium in the genetically heterogeneous PPCD and the absence of these changes in CHED, it remains controversial as to whether these disorders of the posterior cornea are distinct or involve a common aetiological entity. That one variant of PPCD may be related to CHED type 1 is raised by the finding of both disorders in the same family [93] as well as by the fact that CHED type 1 and PPCD have both been mapped to the pericentric region of chromosome 20.

An exciting development is found in the field of in vivo imaging modalities, such as confocal microscopy and spectral domain anterior segment optical coherence tomography. These may be able to help better characterize the corneal dystrophies, certainly those that are unlikely to need surgical excision, and thus add to our knowledge of the clinical manifestations.

Ultimately, the road map between clinical, histopathologic and molecular genetic information about these dystrophies needs to be charted, in order to complete our understanding of these diseases.

References

1 Chiou AG, Florakis GJ, Copeland RL, et al: Recurrent Meesmann's corneal epithelial dystrophy after penetrating keratoplasty. Cornea 1998;17:566–570.

2 Weiss JS, Moeller HU, Lisch W, et al: The IC3D classification of the corneal dystrophies. Cornea 2008;27(suppl 2):S1–S42.

3 Hidayat AA, Risco JM: Amyloidosis of corneal stroma in patients with trachoma. A clinicopathologic study of 62 cases. Ophthalmology 1989;96:1203–1211.

4 Aldave AJ, Principe AH, Lin DY, et al: Lattice dystrophy-like localized amyloidosis of the cornea secondary to trichiasis. Cornea 2005;24:112–115.

5 Robin AL, Green WR, Lapsa TP, et al: Recurrence of macular corneal dystrophy after lamellar keratoplasty. Am J Ophthalmol 1977;84:457–461.

6 Weiss JS, Orlando F, Albert DM: The usefulness of routine alcian blue staining of corneal specimens. Cornea 1988;7:127–132.

7 Bourne WM, Johnson DH, Campbell RJ, et al: The ultrastructure of Descemet's membrane. 3. Fuchs' dystrophy. Arch Ophthalmol 1982;100:1952–1955.

8 Sornson ET: Granular dystrophy of the cornea: an electron microscopic study. Am J Ophthalmol 1965;59:1001–1007.

9 Teng CC: Macular dystrophy of the cornea. A histochemical and electron microscopic study. Am J Ophthalmol 1966;62:436–454.

10 Griffith DG, Fine BS: Light and electron microscopic observations in a superficial corneal dystrophy probable early Reis-Bucklers' type. Am J Ophthalmol 1967;63:1659–1666.

11 Brownstein S, Fine BS, Sherman ME, Zimmerman LE: Granular dystrophy of the cornea. Light and electron microscopic confirmation of recurrence in a graft. Am J Ophthalmol 1974;77:701–710.
12 Dark AJ: Cogan's microcystic dystrophy of the cornea: ultrastructure and photomicroscopy. Br J Ophthalmol 1978;62:821–830.
13 Dark AJ: Bleb dystrophy of the cornea: histochemistry and ultrastructure. Br J Ophthalmol 1977;61: 65–69.
14 Suveges IM: Contribution to the histochemistry of lattice dystrophy of the cornea. Am J Ophthalmol 1967;64:761–766.
15 Garner A: Histochemistry of corneal macular dystrophy. Invest Ophthalmol 1969;8:475–483.
16 Garner A: Histochemistry of corneal granular dystrophy. Br J Ophthalmol 1969;53:799–807.
17 Mustonen RK, McDonald MB, Srivannaboon S, et al: In vivo confocal microscopy of Fuchs' endothelial dystrophy. Cornea 1998;17:493–503.
18 Hernandez-Quintela E, Mayer F, Dighiero P, et al: Confocal microscopy of cystic disorders of the corneal epithelium. Ophthalmology 1998;105: 631–636.
19 Fogle JA, Kenyon KR, Stark WJ, Green WR: Defective epithelial adhesion in anterior corneal dystrophies. Am J Ophthalmol 1975;79:925–940.
20 Guerry D 3rd: Observations on Cogan's microcystic dystrophy of the corneal epithelium. Trans Am Ophthalmol Soc 1965;63:320–334.
21 Cogan DG, Donaldson DD, Kuwabara T, Marshall D: Microcystic dystrophy of the corneal epithelium. Trans Am Ophthalmol Soc 1964;62:213–225.
22 Brodrick JD: Anterior membrane dystrophy following cataract extraction. Br J Ophthalmol 1979;63: 331–335.
23 Aldave AJ, Lin DY, Principe AH, et al: Anterior basement membrane corneal dystrophy and pseudo-unilateral lattice corneal dystrophy in a patient with recurrent corneal erosions. Am J Ophthalmol 2004;137:1124–1127.
24 Cursiefen C, Küchle M, Naumann GO: Changing indications for penetrating keratoplasty: histopathology of 1,250 corneal buttons. Cornea 1998;17:468–470.
25 Rodrigues MM, Fine BS, Laibson PR, et al: Disorders of the corneal epithelium. A clinicopathological study of dot, geographic and fingerprint patterns. Arch Ophthalmol 1974;92:475–82.
26 Guerry D 3rd: Observations on Cogan's microcystic dystrophy of the corneal epithelium. Am J Ophthalmol 1966;62:65–73.
27 Keay L, Jalbert I, Sweeney D, et al: Microcysts: clinical significance and differential diagnosis. Optometry 2001;72:452–460.
28 Bozkurt B, Irkek M: In vivo laser confocal microscopic findings in patients with epithelial basement membrane dystrophy. Eur J Ophthalmol 2009;19: 348–354.
29 Swensson O, Swensson B, Nölle B, et al: Keratin-Gen-Mutationen als Ursache der Epitheldystrophie Meesmann-Wilke und autosomal dominanter Verhornungsstörungen der Haut. Klin Monatsbl Augenheilkd 2000;217:43–51.
30 Patel DV, Grupcheva CN, McGhee CN: Imaging the microstructural abnormalities of Meesmann corneal dystrophy by in vivo confocal microscopy. Cornea 2005;24:669–673.
31 Alvarez-Fischer M, Alvarez de Toledo J, Barraquer RI: Lisch corneal dystrophy. Cornea 2005;24: 494–495.
32 Wessel MM, Sarkar JS, Jakobiec FA, et al: Treatment of Lisch corneal dystrophy with photorefractive keratectomy and mitomycin C. Cornea, E-pub ahead of print.
33 Li S, Edward DP, Ratnakar KS, et al: Clinicohistopathological findings of gelatinous drop-like corneal dystrophy among Asians. Cornea 1996;15: 355–362.
34 Vemuganti GK, Sridhar MS, Edward DP, Sing S, et al: Subepithelial amyloid deposits in congenital hereditary endothelial dystrophy: a histopathologic study of five cases. Cornea 2002;21:524–529.
35 Jing Y, Liu C, Wang L: A novel TACSTD2 mutation identified in two Chinese brothers with gelatinous drop-like corneal dystrophy. Mol Vis 2009;15: 1580–1588.
36 Ridgway AE, Akhtar S, Munier FL, et al: Ultrastructural and molecular analysis of Bowman's layer corneal dystrophies: an epithelial origin? Invest Ophthalmol Vis Sci 2000;41:3286–3292.
37 Akhtar S, Bron AJ, Qin X, et al: Gelatinous drop-like corneal dystrophy in a child with developmental delay: clinicopathological features and exclusion of the M1S1 gene. Eye 2005;19:198–204.
38 Takaoka M, Nakamura T, Ban Y, et al: Phenotypic investigation of cell junction-related proteins in gelatinous drop-like corneal dystrophy. Invest Ophthalmol Vis Sci 2007;48:1095–1101.
39 Kinoshita S, Nishida K, Duta A, et al: Epithelial barrier function and ultrastructure of gelatinous drop-like corneal dystrophy. Cornea 2000;19:551–555.
40 Yoshida S, Kumano Y, Yoshida A, et al: Two brothers with gelatinous drop-like dystrophy at different stages of the disease: role of mutational analysis. Am J Ophthalmol 2002;133:830–832.
41 Akiya S, Takahashi H, Furukawa H, et al: A case of one eye with gelatinous drop-like corneal dystrophy and the other eye with band-shaped spheroidal corneal degeneration. Ophthalmologica 1995;209: 96–100.

42 Quantock AJ, Nishida K, Kinoshita S: Histopathology of recurrent gelatinous drop-like corneal dystrophy. Cornea 1998;17:215–221.
43 Buchi ER, Daicker B, Uffer S, Gudat F: Primary gelatinous drop-like corneal dystrophy in a white woman. A pathologic, ultrastructural, and immunohistochemical study. Cornea 1994;13:190–194.
44 Perez-Santonja JJ, Galal A, Cardona C, et al: Severe corneal epithelial sloughing during laser in situ keratomileusis as a presenting sign for silent epithelial basement membrane dystrophy. J Cataract Refract Surg 2005;31:1932–1937.
45 Akiya S, Furukawa H, Sakamoto H, et al: Histopathologic and immunohistochemical findings in gelatinous drop-like corneal dystrophy. Ophthalmic Res 1990;22:371–376.
46 Ohnishi Y, Shinoda Y, Ishibashi T, et al: The origin of amyloid in gelatinous drop-like corneal dystrophy. Curr Eye Res 1982;2:225–231.
47 Küchle M, Green WR, Völcker H, et al: Reevaluation of corneal dystrophies of Bowman's layer and the anterior stroma (Reis-Bücklers and Thiel-Behnke types): a light and electron microscopic study of eight corneas and a review of the literature. Cornea 1995;14:333–354.
48 Aldave AJ, Rayner SA, King JA, et al: A unique corneal dystrophy of Bowman's layer and stroma associated with the Gly623Asp mutation in the transforming growth factor beta-induced (TGFBI) gene. Ophthalmology 2005;112:1017–1022.
49 Werner LP, Werner L, Dighiero P, et al: Confocal microscopy in Bowman and stromal corneal dystrophies. Ophthalmology 1999;106:1697–1704.
50 Kurome H, Noda S, Hayasaka S, Setogawa T: A Japanese family with Grayson-Wilbrandt variant of Reis-Bücklers' corneal dystrophy. Jpn J Ophthalmol 1993;37:143–147.
51 Grayson M, Wilbrandt H: Dystrophy of the anterior limiting membrane of the cornea (Reis-Bücklers' type). Am J Ophthalmol 1966;61:345–349.
52 Stuart JC, Mund ML, Iwamoto T, et al: Recurrent granular corneal dystrophy. Am J Ophthalmol 1975;79:18–24.
53 Rodrigues MM, Streeten BW, Krachmer JH, et al: Microfibrillar protein and phospholipid in granular corneal dystrophy. Arch Ophthalmol 1983;101:802–810.
54 Johnson BL, Brown SI, Zaidman GW: A light and electron microscopic study of recurrent granular dystrophy of the cornea. Am J Ophthalmol 1981;92:49–58.
55 Choi SI, Kim TI, Kim KS, et al: Decreased catalase expression and increased susceptibility to oxidative stress in primary cultured corneal fibroblasts from patients with granular corneal dystrophy type II. Am J Pathol 2009;175:248–261.
56 Nemeth G, Felszeghy S, Kenyeres A, et al: Cell adhesion molecules in stromal corneal dystrophies. Histol Histopathol 2008;23:945–952.
57 Kaluzny BJ, Szkulmowska A, Szkulmomski M, et al: Granular corneal dystrophy in 830-nm spectral optical coherence tomography. Cornea 2008;27:830–832.
58 Akhtar S, Meek KM, Ridgway AE, et al: Deposits and proteoglycan changes in primary and recurrent granular dystrophy of the cornea. Arch Ophthalmol 1999;117:310–321.
59 Klintworth GK, Smith CF: Acridine orange particles in cultured fibroblasts. A comparative study of macular corneal dystrophy, systemic mucopolysaccharidoses types I-H and II, and normal controls. Arch Pathol Lab Med 1979;103:297–299.
60 Cursiefen C, Hofmann-Rummelt C, Schlötzer-Schrehardt U, et al: Immunophenotype classification of macular corneal dystrophy: first case report of immunophenotype I A outside of Saudi Arabia. A clinical histopathological correlation with immunohistochemistry and electron microscopy. Klin Monatsbl Augenheilkd 2000;217:118–126.
61 Sultana A, Klintworth GK, Thonar EJ, Vemuganti GK, Kannabiran C: Immunophenotypes of macular corneal dystrophy in India and correlation with mutations in CHST6. Mol Vis 2009;15:319–325.
62 Edward DP, Yue BY, Sugar J, et al: Heterogeneity in macular corneal dystrophy. Arch Ophthalmol 1988;106:1579–1583.
63 Hori S, et al: Transmission and scanning electron microscopic studies on endothelial cells in macular corneal dystrophy. Jpn J Ophthalmol 1982;26:190–198.
64 Funderburgh JL, Funderburgh ML, Rodrigues MM, et al: Altered antigenicity of keratan sulfate proteoglycan in selected corneal diseases. Invest Ophthalmol Vis Sci 1990;31:419–428.
65 Jonasson F, Jonasson JH, Garner A, Rice NS: Macular corneal dystrophy in Iceland. Eye (Lond) 1989;3:446–454.
66 Aldave AJ, Yellore VS, Somnez B, et al: A novel variant of combined granular-lattice corneal dystrophy associated with the Met619Lys mutation in the TGFBI gene. Arch Ophthalmol 2008;126:371–377.
67 Awwad ST, Di Pascuale MA, Hogan RN, et al: Avellino corneal dystrophy worsening after laser in situ keratomileusis: further clinicopathologic observations and proposed pathogenesis. Am J Ophthalmol 2008;145:656–661.
68 Ferry AP, Benson WH, Weinberg RS: Combined granular-lattice ('Avellino') corneal dystrophy. Trans Am Ophthalmol Soc 1997;95:61–77.
69 Karp CL, Scott IU, Green WR, et al: Central cloudy corneal dystrophy of Francois. A clinicopathologic study. Arch Ophthalmol 1997;115:1058–1062.

70 Nicholson DH, Green WR, Cross HE, et al: A clinical and histopathological study of Francois-Neetens speckled corneal dystrophy. Am J Ophthalmol 1977; 83:554–560.

71 Banning CS, Larson PM, Randleman JB: Outcome of LASIK in fleck corneal dystrophy. Cornea 2006; 25:1262–1264.

72 Holopainen JM, Moilanen JAO, Tervo TMT: In vivo confocal microscopy of Fleck dystrophy and pre-Descemet's membrane corneal dystrophy. Cornea 2003;22:160–163.

73 Freddo TF, Polack FM, Leibowitz HM: Ultrastructural changes in the posterior layers of the cornea in Schnyder's crystalline dystrophy. Cornea 1989;8:170–177.

74 Hoang-Xuan T, Pouliquen Y, Savoldelli M, Gasteau J: Dystrophie cristalline de Schnyder. J Fr Ophtalmol 1985;8:735–742.

75 Yamada M, Mochizuki H, Kamata Y, et al: Quantitative analysis of lipid deposits from Schnyder's corneal dystrophy. Br J Ophthalmol 1998;82:444–447.

76 Gaynor PM, Zhang WY, Weiss JS, et al: Accumulation of HDL apolipoproteins accompanies abnormal cholesterol accumulation in Schnyder's corneal dystrophy. Arterioscler Thromb Vasc Biol 1996;16: 992–999.

77 Ciancaglini M, Carpineto P, Zuppardi E, et al: Morphological evaluation of Schnyder's central crystalline dystrophy by confocal microscopy before and after phototherapeutic keratectomy. J Cataract Refract Surg 2001;27:1892–1895.

78 Brooks AM, Grant G, Gillies WE: A comparison of corneal endothelial morphology in cornea guttata, Fuchs' dystrophy and bullous keratopathy. Aust NZ J Ophthalmol 1988;16:93–100.

79 Kenney MC, et al: Altered expression of aquaporins in bullous keratopathy and Fuchs' dystrophy corneas. J Histochem Cytochem 2004;52:1341–1350.

80 Bergmanson JP, Sheldon TM, Goosey JD: Fuchs' endothelial dystrophy: a fresh look at an aging disease. Ophthalmic Physiol Opt 1999;19:210–222.

81 Borderie VM, Baudrimont M, Vallée A, et al: Corneal endothelial cell apoptosis in patients with Fuchs' dystrophy. Invest Ophthalmol Vis Sci 2000; 41:2501–2505.

82 Ljubimov AV, Atilano RS, Garner MH, et al: Extracellular matrix and Na^+,K^+-ATPase in human corneas following cataract surgery: comparison with bullous keratopathy and Fuchs' dystrophy corneas. Cornea 2002;21:74–80.

83 Renard G, Petroutsos G, Savoldelli M, Pouliquen Y: Polymorphic posterior corneal dystrophy. Histological and ultrastructural study of 2 cases. J Fr Ophtalmol 1983;6:7–23.

84 Richardson WP, Hettinger ME: Endothelial and epithelial-like cell formations in a case of posterior polymorphous dystrophy. Arch Ophthalmol 1985; 103:1520–1524.

85 Feil SH, Barraquer J, Howell DN, et al: Extrusion of abnormal endothelium into the posterior corneal stroma in a patient with posterior polymorphous dystrophy. Cornea 1997;16:439–446.

86 Jirsova K, Merjava S, Martincova R, et al: Immunohistochemical characterization of cytokeratins in the abnormal corneal endothelium of posterior polymorphous corneal dystrophy patients. Exp Eye Res 2007;84:680–686.

87 Cheng LL, Young AL, Wong AK, et al: Confocal microscopy of posterior polymorphous endothelial dystrophy. Cornea 2005;24:599–602.

88 Boruchoff SA, Weiner MJ, Albert DM: Recurrence of posterior polymorphous corneal dystrophy after penetrating keratoplasty. Am J Ophthalmol 1990; 109:323–328.

89 Cibis GW, Tripathi RC: The differential diagnosis of Descemet's tears (Haab's striae) and posterior polymorpous dystrophy bands. A clinicopathologic study. Ophthalmology 1982;89:614–620.

90 Ehlers N, Modis L, Moller-Pedersen T: A morphological and functional study of Congenital Hereditary Endothelial Dystrophy. Acta Ophthalmol Scand 1998;76:314–318.

91 Mahmood MA, Teichmann KD: Corneal amyloidosis associated with congenital hereditary endothelial dystrophy. Cornea 2000;19:570–573.

92 Cockerham GC, Laver NV, Hidayat AA, et al: An immunohistochemical analysis and comparison of posterior polymorphous dystrophy with congenital hereditary endothelial dystrophy. Cornea 2002;21: 787–791.

93 Cibis GW, Krachmer JA, Phelps CD, et al: The clinical spectrum of posterior polymorphous dystrophy. Arch Ophthalmol 1977;95:1529–1537.

Geeta K. Vemuganti, MD, DNB, FNAMS
School of Medical Sciences
University of Hyderabad
Hyderabad, 500046 (India)
Tel. +91 40 2301 3279/2301 4781, E-Mail gkvemuganti@gmail.com

Lisch W, Seitz B (eds): Corneal Dystrophies.
Dev Ophthalmol. Basel, Karger, 2011, vol 48, pp 51–66

The Genetics of the Corneal Dystrophies

Anthony J. Aldave

The Jules Stein Eye Institute, David Geffen School of Medicine, The University of California, Los Angeles, Calif., USA

Abstract

Several comprehensive reviews have been written recently that summarize what is currently known about the molecular genetic basis of the corneal dystrophies. The one that is the current definitive reference on the subject is the IC3D classification of the corneal dystrophies, written by an international group of experts on the corneal dystrophies. In this work, each gene in which a pathogenic mutation has been identified in a patient with a corneal dystrophy is listed and an appendix is provided with a complete list of the genes and the mutations listed at the nucleotide and amino acid levels (with references). As the IC3D classification of the corneal dystrophies is readily available to the reader both in print and online, this chapter will not focus on reviewing the genes and mutations that have been associated with the corneal dystrophies. Instead, it will provide an overview of the genetics of the corneal dystrophies, discussing first the clinical and genetic spectrum of the corneal dystrophies and then the limitations of a genetically based classification system for the corneal dystrophies. The last section of this chapter will discuss how the discovery of mutations that cause the corneal dystrophies is not the end of the process of scientific discovery, but only the beginning, as vision scientists attempt to determine how the identified mutations lead to the formation of corneal deposits or loss of endothelial function, and develop strategies to modulate gene expression.

Several comprehensive reviews have been written recently that summarize what is currently known about the molecular genetic basis of the corneal dystrophies [1, 2]. The one that is the current definitive reference on the subject is the IC3D classification of the corneal dystrophies, written by an international group of experts on the corneal dystrophies [2]. In this work, each gene in which a pathogenic mutation has been identified in a patient with a corneal dystrophy is listed and an appendix is provided with a complete list of the genes and the mutations listed at the nucleotide and amino acid levels (with references). As the IC3D classification of the corneal dystrophies is readily available to the reader both in print and online (www.corneasociety.org/ic3d), and another chapter in this book is devoted to reviewing this collaborative work, this chapter will not focus on reviewing the genes and mutations that have been associated with the corneal dystrophies. Instead, it will provide an overview of the genetics of the corneal dystrophies, discussing first the clinical and genetic spectrum of the corneal dystrophies and then the limitations of a genetically based classification system for the corneal dystrophies. The last section of this chapter will discuss how the discovery of mutations that cause the corneal dystrophies is not the end of the process of scientific discovery, but only the beginning, as vision scientists attempt to determine how the identified mutations lead to the formation of corneal deposits or loss of endothelial function, and develop strategies to modulate gene expression.

The Genetic and Clinical Spectrum of the Corneal Dystrophies

Although the corneal dystrophies are a heterogeneous group of inherited corneal disorders, generalizations can be made about the clinical and genetic spectrum of these disorders.

Inheritance

With a few notable exceptions, the corneal dystrophies are inherited in an autosomal dominant manner, following simple mendelian inheritance. Exceptions to this include the corneal dystrophies that are inherited in an autosomal recessive manner, such as macular corneal dystrophy (MIM No. 217800) and autosomal recessive congenital hereditary endothelial dystrophy (CHED2, MIM No. 217700), and those inherited in an X-linked recessive manner, such as Lisch epithelial corneal dystrophy and X-linked endothelial corneal dystrophy. In addition, several reports in the literature have documented the occurrence of a dominantly inherited corneal dystrophy in an individual born to unaffected parents. Identification of the pathogenic mutation in the affected individual but not in either of the individual's parents raised the possibility of mistaken parentage, which was excluded based on confirmatory maternity and paternity testing [3–5]. In addition to these reports of spontaneous mutations in the transforming growth factor, β-induced gene (*TGFBI,* MIM No. 601692) causing the development of a dominantly inherited corneal dystrophy in a family with no other affected members, uniparental disomy has been reported as a cause of macular corneal dystrophy in an affected individual found to be homozygous for a mutant allele in the carbohydrate sulfotransferase 6 gene (*CHST6,* MIM No. 605294) that was present in the heterozygous state in his mother and absent in his father [6]. While it is very likely that other unreported cases of dominant corneal dystrophies secondary to spontaneous mutations and recessive corneal dystrophies secondary to uniparental disomy exist, they undoubtedly represent a small minority of all cases of dominant and recessive corneal dystrophies. Therefore, obtaining a family history of other affected individuals or of consanguinity is typically of value when questioning an individual with a dominantly or recessively inherited corneal dystrophy, respectively.

Pathogenesis

Single Gene Disorder versus Locus Heterogeneity

The majority of the corneal dystrophies are single gene disorders, in which coding region mutations in a single gene are associated with a particular dystrophy. However, locus heterogeneity, in which mutations in 2 or more genes mapped to different chromosomal loci are responsible for producing the same affected phenotype, has been demonstrated for 2 different corneal dystrophies, i.e. Meesmann corneal dystrophy (MIM No. 122100) and posterior polymorphous corneal dystrophy (PPCD1, MIM No. 122000; PPCD2, MIM No. 609140; PPCD3, MIM No. 609141). Meesmann corneal dystrophy is associated with mutations in 2 different genes, keratin 3 (*KRT3,* MIM No. 148043) and keratin 12 (*KRT12,* MIM No. 601687), located on chromosomes 12 and 17, respectively. As the expression of these genes is limited to the cornea, so is the affected phenotype [7]. While the majority of the reported mutations have been identified in *KRT12,* the affected phenotype associated with the reported *KRT3* mutations is not distinguishable from the clinical appearance and course associated with *KRT12* mutations [2]. Similarly, mutations identified in the zinc finger E-box binding homeobox 1 gene (*ZEB1,* MIM No. 189909) on chromosome 10 have been associated with a phenotype range of PPCD that cannot be distinguished from that seen in affected individuals in families linked to the PPCD1 locus on chromosome 20 [8–12]. To date, 22 coding region mutations have been identified in the *ZEB1* gene in 59 PPCD probands that have been screened, indicating that PPCD3 accounts for approximately 30–40% of all PPCD cases [Pham MN, et al.: IOVS 2009;50:E-abstract 5500; 9, 11–13]. It is unknown what percentage of the remaining pedigrees represents PPCD1, as only a handful of families have been of sufficient size to perform either a genome-wide linkage analysis or a chromosome 20 linkage replication study. It is possible that some of the families in which *ZEB1* mutations were not identified still represent PPCD3, associated with non-coding region mutations. It is also possible that some of the families in which *ZEB1* mutations were not identified represent PPCD2, associated with mutations in the collagen, type VIII, α-2 gene (*COL8A2,* MIM No. 120252) [14, 15], although the limited evidence supporting the PPCD2 locus, and in light of the fact that linkage has never been demonstrated for PPCD to the *COL8A2* locus on chromosome 1, has led to questions regarding whether *COL8A2* mutations are involved in PPCD [16].

Gain of Function versus Loss of Function

The majority of the corneal dystrophies are dominantly inherited disorders that are caused by mutations in genes coding for a structural protein. Mutations in these genes result in the formation of abnormal protein products that have altered characteristics when compared to the wild-type protein product. These altered characteristics may result in abnormal protein aggregation or novel interactions with other components of the cornea, which lead to loss of corneal clarity. This process, known as a gain of function, is exemplified by the TGFBI dystrophies, in which *TGBFI* mutations lead to the formation of aggregates of the TGFBI protein (TGFBIp) in the Bowman layer and stroma that cause loss of corneal clarity. In these dystrophies, TGBFIp, which is expressed by the corneal epithelial cells and keratocytes, takes on novel functions (or most appropriately novel dysfunctions) in the cornea.

In contrast, the recessively inherited corneal dystrophies are associated with mutations in genes encoding enzymatic proteins, which result in loss of protein function. If the wild-type protein product is necessary to maintain corneal clarity, its loss may result in stromal opacification, as in macular corneal dystrophy, or stromal edema, as is seen in CHED.

Penetrance

The dominantly inherited corneal dystrophies have long been assumed to be fully penetrant disorders, meaning that any individual who inherits a pathogenic mutation will demonstrate the affected phenotype. Thus, penetrance is an all or nothing phenomenon in an individual, as opposed to expressivity, which is a measure of the degree to which the affected phenotype is manifest in an individual. Although complete penetrance is often assumed in the setting of parameters for linkage analysis to identify the genetic loci associated with the corneal dystrophies, the authors have identified 2 PPCD pedigrees in which the parents of affected individuals have been found to be clinically unaffected. As *ZEB1* coding region mutations were not identified in the affected proband from each of these families, we did not perform genetic screening in the clinically unaffected parents and thus are not able to definitively state that these individuals demonstrate incomplete penetrance. The presence of 2 affected offspring in 1 of these families effectively excludes the possibility of a spontaneous mutation or mistaken paternity, although germ line mosaicism remains a possible explanation. Incomplete penetrance has been confirmed in another PPCD family, which was the family used to map PPCD to chromosome 10 and in which *ZEB1* mutations were first identified in association with PPCD3 [11].

Localization of Expression

One of the long-held dicta regarding the corneal dystrophies is that expression of the affected phenotype is limited to the cornea. Indeed, it has been confirmed that in the TGBFI dystrophies, the dystrophic deposits are confined to the cornea, and are not present in any extraocular tissues [17]. Various theories have been put forth to explain this observation, the most plausible of which is that the avascularity of the cornea allows the formation of dystrophic deposits that would be cleared away by blood-borne molecular scavengers in other tissues. In support of this theory are the observations that dystrophic corneal deposits rarely involve the peripheral cornea, near the limbal vessels, and that dystrophic deposits are not present in areas of corneal vascularization associated with pterygium formation or phthisis bulbi [18]. However, a number of different corneal dystrophies have been associated with extracorneal manifestations, such as absent or low levels of serum keratan sulfate in patients with macular corneal dystrophy [19], abdominal wall hernia formation in patients with PPCD3 [9, 11], and elevated serum cholesterol levels [20] and abnormal cholesterol metabolism in skin fibroblasts [21] in patients with Schnyder corneal dystrophy (MIM No. 121800).

Expressivity

Many of the corneal dystrophies demonstrate a great degree of heterogeneity when one considers the range of phenotypes that are seen in affected individuals who demonstrate the same genotype, which is known as expressivity. When comparing the range of phenotypes manifest in 2 different families with the same corneal dystrophy associated with the same mutant allele, one would expect some degree of interfamilial variability due to the differences in the genetic background and environmental exposures of the 2 families. However, significant differences in expressivity of some corneal dystrophies, such as the TGFBI dystrophies, have been described even in affected siblings that carry the same mutant allele, have similar genetic backgrounds and have been exposed to the same environmental factors [22] (fig. 1). In other dystrophies, such as PPCD, expressivity can vary significantly in regard to the onset of the affected phenotype, with affected members of a family possessing the same mutant allele demonstrating either congenital corneal edema, corneal edema presenting later in life, or remaining asymptomatic [9, 23]. Similarly, the familiar dictum that the corneal deposits that characterize the corneal dystrophies are typically bilateral and symmetrically distributed in a given patient has been challenged by the multiple reports of patients with unilateral corneal dystrophies [24–27]. Thus, the interfamilial, intrafamilial and interocular expressivity observed between families, within families and between the 2 eyes of an affected individual with the same pathogenic mutation, respectively, indicates that the affected phenotype may be determined by local factors that remain to be elucidated.

Genotype-Phenotype Associations

For the majority of the corneal dystrophies, a genotype-phenotype correlation has not been demonstrated, in that multiple different identified coding region mutations

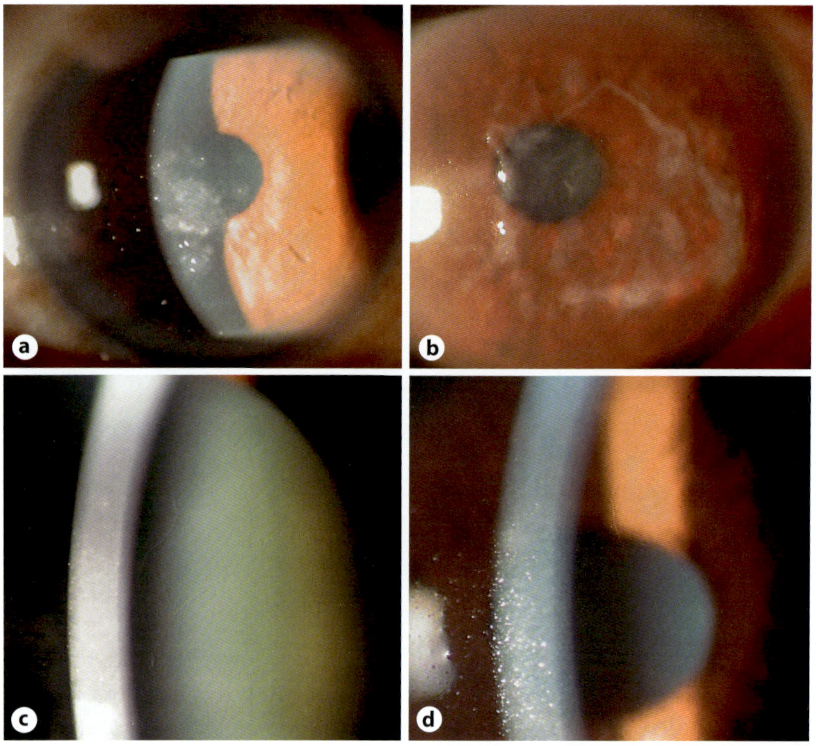

Fig. 1. Intrafamilial phenotypic heterogeneity. Slit lamp photomicrographs of the corneal findings in 4 siblings with a suspected TGBFI dystrophy. While 2 of the siblings demonstrated subepithelial and Bowman layer opacities (**a, b**), consistent with a Bowman layer dystrophy, 2 other siblings demonstrated stromal lattice lines (**c, d**), consistent with classic lattice corneal dystrophy. Screening of *TGBFI* revealed a novel Gly623Asp mutation that segregated with the affected phenotype in the family [22]. Bottom right photo (**d**) reproduced by permission of *Ophthalmology*.

are associated with overlapping clinical features [1, 2]. Thus, none of the more than 120 mutations identified to date in *CHST6* in patients with macular corneal dystrophy and none of the 48 mutations identified in the solute carrier family 4, member 11 gene (*SLC4A11,* MIM No. 610206) in patients with autosomal recessive CHED is associated with a reproducibly distinct phenotype [2]. However, for a few of the corneal dystrophies, such as the dystrophies associated with mutations in TGFBI, a general phenotype-genotype correlation is evident. Mutations in codons 124 and 555 in *TGFBI* are associated with each of the classic TGFBI dystrophies, with variant clinical forms associated with a number of uncommon mutations scattered across 5 of the gene's 17 exons [2]. Each of the commonly encountered mutations is associated with a characteristic phenotype, so that one may predict the eventual phenotype and clinical course of an individual identified with the mutation during presymptomatic screening. As mentioned previously, variability in the expressivity of the affected phenotype may be seen, but in the author's experience this is more common with the variant

TGFBI dystrophies. The clustering of pathogenic mutations in 2 hotspots in *TGFBI*, and the observed phenotype-genotype correlation for the classic TGBFI dystrophies makes diagnostic screening of *TGFBI* a useful clinical tool for the clinician looking to confirm or refute a presumptive clinical diagnosis [1, 28].

Genetic Classification of the Corneal Dystrophies

Even though the genetic basis for the majority of the corneal dystrophies has been identified, the IC3D classification is still organized by the anatomic level of involvement for reasons that are expounded upon in the chapter in this book that is devoted to reviewing this collaborative work.

Benefits of an Anatomically Based Classification System

In essence, if a classification system is being devised to serve as a resource to clinicians to facilitate accurate diagnosis, understanding and management of the corneal dystrophies, it should be organized in a format that is 'clinician-friendly'. Therefore, the framework of such a classification system should be based on characteristic features of the corneal dystrophies that allow them to be differentiated from one another, as well as nondystrophic corneal disorders. As there is significant age-dependent variability in the degree of corneal edema or the number and morphology of the opacities that characterize many of the corneal dystrophies, reliance upon diagnosing and classifying the corneal dystrophies based upon these characteristics is problematic. Much more consistent is the anatomic level of the cornea that is involved in each corneal dystrophy, which can be readily assessed by the clinician at the slit lamp. Although this is perhaps the most clinician-friendly system, it is not without its own limitations as well. Clinicians are quick to recognize that bilateral epithelial and/or stromal edema in a patient without a history of prior intraocular surgery is likely due to an endothelial dystrophy. Thus, the endothelial dystrophies typically produce visual impairment not through abnormalities in the endothelium or Descemet membrane, but instead in the epithelium and stroma. Additionally, ample evidence exists to support the belief that the majority of the dysfunctional TGBFIp that accumulates in the Bowman layer or stroma in patients affected with a TGFBI dystrophy is actually of an epithelial genesis [29, 30]. This evidence is consistent with observations made by clinicians that recurrences of the TGFBI dystrophies following penetrating or deep anterior lamellar keratoplasty, or following laser phototherapeutic keratectomy, are typically very superficial, and with time extend to involve the corneal stroma (fig. 2). Similarly, examination of young patients with granular, lattice or combined granular-lattice corneal dystrophy (granular corneal dystrophy, type 2) will typically demonstrate deposits that first appear in the subepithelial region. Therefore, although the

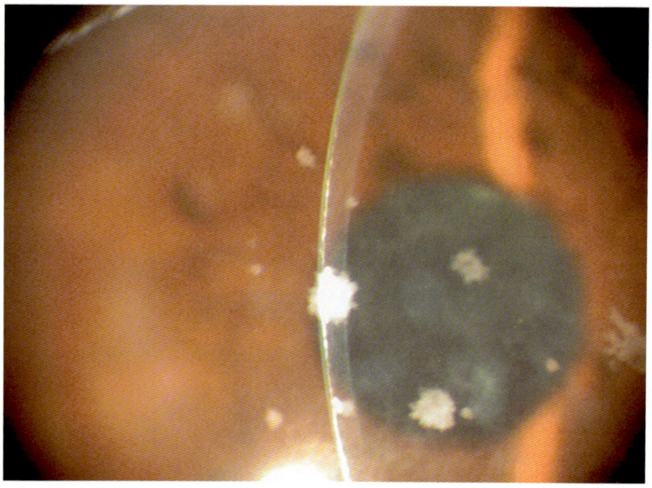

Fig. 2. Recurrence of granular corneal dystrophy, type 2, following phototherapeutic keratectomy. Slit lamp photomicrograph demonstrating superficial opacification that developed several years after phototherapeutic keratectomy was performed. The superficial nature of the recurrence suggests an epithelial source for the recurrent TGFBI protein. Screening of *TGFBI* in the patient revealed the Arg124His mutation associated with granular corneal dystrophy, type 2.

deposits that the clinician observes in TGFBI dystrophies are located in the Bowman layer and stroma, thus leading to their classification as Bowman layer and stromal dystrophies, they are likely primarily of an epithelial origin.

Disadvantages of a Genetically Based Classification System

Although many vision science researchers and geneticists would likely be in favor of a genetically based classification system for the corneal dystrophies, such a system would have significant limitations, both now and in the future.

The Genetic Basis of Many of the Corneal Dystrophies Remains Unknown

In a seminal article published in 1994, Dr. Stone et al. [31] demonstrated linkage of granular, lattice and combined granular-lattice corneal dystrophies to chromosome 5q. Three years later, Munier et al. [32] identified mutations in what is now known as the *TGFBI* gene in families with each of these 3 dystrophies, as well as Reis-Bücklers corneal dystrophy. In the following decade, the genetic basis of many of the most common corneal dystrophies has been discovered, although the basis of some of the most common, including classic Fuchs corneal dystrophy, await discovery [1, 2]. However, until the discovery of the genetic basis of the corneal dystrophies is complete, it is not possible to create a classification system for the corneal dystrophies based primarily

Table 1. Criteria to support the pathogenicity of an identified coding region variant

- Presence of 2 mutant alleles in an autosomal recessive disorder and 1 mutant allele in an autosomal dominant disorder
- Change in the involved encoded amino acid in the case of a missense mutation
- Formation or loss of a splice site in the case of a silent mutation (synonymous substitution)
- Loss of functional protein domains in the case of a frameshift or nonsense mutation
- Segregation with the affected phenotype in the identified pedigree
- Absence of the identified variant in a suitable number of unaffected, unrelated individuals (typically >100)
- Evolutionary conservation of the involved amino acid in the case of a missense mutation
- Functional analysis of the identified variant demonstrating an alteration in the structure, localization or function of the encoded protein

on the mutated gene or gene product. In addition, even for those dystrophies for which strong evidence exists to support the pathogenicity of the mutations identified in the involved gene(s), not all affected probands possess a disease-causing mutation. In the case of autosomal recessive CHED, *SLC4A11* coding region mutations have been identified in 82% (76 of 93) of probands [33–41] and in the case of PPCD, *ZEB1* coding region mutations have been identified in only 37% (22 of 59) of probands [Pham MN, et al.: IOVS 2009;50:E-abstract 5500; 9, 11–13]. Multiple explanations exist for the failure to observe coding region mutations in a significant percentage of patients with these and other corneal dystrophies, including: locus heterogeneity (as in the case of posterior polymorphous corneal dystrophy); phenocopy (a phenotype that may be misdiagnosed as a given inherited disorder associated with a particular genotype); pathogenic noncoding mutations [which have been reported previously in individuals with fleck corneal dystrophy (MIM No. 121850) and autosomal recessive CHED] [34, 38, 42], and deletion of a portion or all of the coding region or alteration in a PCR primer binding site. Therefore, a sufficient number of questions remain regarding the genetic basis of many of the corneal dystrophies, even those for which pathogenic mutations have been identified, to significantly impair the ability of a genetically based system to accurately and comprehensively classify the corneal dystrophies.

Lack of Consensus Regarding Criteria to Determine Pathogenicity of Identified Mutations

It is generally accepted that for an identified coding region variant to be considered pathogenic, several criteria should be met, as shown in table 1.

However, a review of the corneal dystrophy literature demonstrates that for most of the reported presumed pathogenic mutations, one or more of the criteria in table 1 have not been met. In fact, functional analysis to confirm the pathogenicity of an identified sequence variant has been performed for a very small minority of the mutations that have been identified to date in association with a corneal dystrophy. In the absence of functional investigations, the other criteria to support the probable pathogenicity of an identified mutation are all that may be relied upon. Therefore, when a sequence variant is identified in a candidate gene for a given corneal dystrophy (for which the genetic basis is not yet known), the inability or failure to demonstrate segregation of the mutation with the affected phenotype will inevitably lead to disagreement about the validity of the identified variant. In such situations, the demonstration or exclusion of linkage of the dystrophy to the proposed genetic locus, and the screening of the involved gene in a large number of unrelated, affected probands with the same corneal dystrophy are effective means to provide additional evidence for or against the pathogenicity of the proposed mutation(s) [43–45]. It should be kept in mind that even nonsense mutations, which typically produce a truncated, nonfunctional protein product, may not always be disease causing, and even if they are, they may not be responsible for the disease under investigation [46–49]. Such varying levels of evidence to support the involvement of coding region mutations in various genes is particularly evident in the corneal endothelial dystrophies, with disagreement among corneal dystrophy experts on the role of the visual system homeobox 1 gene (*VSX1*, MIM No. 605020) in PPCD1 [44, 45, 50–52], *COL8A2* in PPCD2 and Fuchs corneal dystrophy [14–16, 43, 53, 54], and *SLC4A11* in Fuchs corneal dystrophy [55]. Until an agreement can be reached on whether these genes do or do not play a role in each of these corneal dystrophies, a consensus will not be reached on a genetically based classification system.

Moving beyond the Mutation: Understanding the Genes That Control Corneal Clarity and Developing Strategies to Modulate Gene Expression

While the identification of the genetic basis of the corneal dystrophies through linkage and association analyses has provided clinicians with an additional clinical tool to confirm or refute presumptive clinical diagnoses, it is not the end, but instead the beginning of the process of scientific discovery. The identification of the genes that play a role in the maintenance of corneal clarity leads not only to new avenues of investigation for vision scientists, but also molecular targets for the development of gene-based therapeutic strategies.

The Genetic Basis for the Maintenance of Corneal Clarity

The search for the genes that cause various corneal dystrophies may start with knowledge about the role that the disease gene likely plays in the cornea, as was the case for macular corneal dystrophy. Dr. Klintworth had identified that this recessive dystrophy was associated with glycosaminoglycan accumulation in the corneas of affected individuals in the mid 1960s [56], and both he and others subsequently identified that this accumulation was associated with an error in the synthesis of keratan sulfate, likely due to a defective sulfotransferase [57, 58]. However, it was not until 2000 that Dr. Akama et al. [59] were able to identify mutations in patients with macular corneal dystrophy in a newly described sulfotransferase gene, *CHST6*. This is in contrast to the search for the genetic basis of autosomal recessive CHED, for which the biochemical basis of the disorder was unknown. When two groups independently identified mutations in the sodium borate cotransporter gene *SCL4A11* in families with autosomal recessive CHED [33, 38], the discovery was met with great surprise as borate had not been previously implicated as playing a role in corneal endothelial cell physiology, and given the well-described role of bicarbonate transport across the corneal endothelium in maintaining corneal transparency [60].

As is the case with NaBC1, the protein product of *SLC4A11*, it is still not clear what role TGFBIp plays in the maintenance of corneal clarity. Based on the presence of 4 FAS-1 domains in TGFBIp, the protein is thought to play a role in mediating adhesion and/or spreading of various cell types [61]. Even less well understood than the role that NaBC1 and TGFBIp play in the maintenance of the clarity and structure of the cornea is the way in which the identified mutations lead to the development of the affected phenotype. Surprisingly, Slc4a11$^{-/-}$ mice do not demonstrate corneal edema and the corneal endothelial cells are morphologically normal [62]. Attempts to create a transgenic knock-in animal model of a TGBFI dystrophy have thus far not been successful in producing a corneal phenotype, leaving researchers to speculate on the mechanisms involved in dystrophic corneal TGFBIp deposition [63].

Genetic Therapy for the Corneal Dystrophies

Why the Cornea Is a Good Model

While several well-published trials of gene-based therapy for inherited retinal disorders in humans and primates have received significant attention in the last several years [64–66], gene-based therapies for inherited corneal disorders remain in the in vitro stage at present. The cornea is an excellent model for genetic therapy for a variety of reasons, as detailed in excellent review articles that have been written on the subject [67, 68]. The accessibility and transparency of the cornea allow for direct observation of the target tissue in live animals to assess the effects of a therapeutic intervention. Obtaining a sample of the epithelium and even stroma to assess such effects at an ultrastructural level is performed much more easily than with other targeted organs, which may require sacrificing the animal. A variety of therapeutic approaches are possible, including topical, intrastromal and intracameral gene delivery or silencing, depending on the targeted cell type and the desired effect on gene expression. In addition, the relatively immune-privileged nature of the eye allows for the use of viral vectors for gene transfer that could not be used in other target tissues because of concerns regarding immunogenicity [67, 69, 70]. The ability to easily transplant a cornea also provides the opportunity for ex vivo gene transfer or modulation in the donor cornea prior to transplantation, with the goal of reducing the immunogenicity or risk of recurrent disease in the donor cornea. In the case of either in vivo or ex vivo genetic modulation, the contralateral eye may serve as a control, facilitating a determination of the effects of the therapeutic intervention [67, 71, 72].

Goals of Genetic Therapy
As mentioned previously, the corneal dystrophies are associated with mutations in genes encoding proteins that result in either a gain or a loss of protein function. In the case of the former, the goal of genetic therapy would be inhibition of protein expression, through methods such as inhibition of activation of the gene promoter, activation of a repressor of gene transcription, or prevention of translation using a technique such as RNA interference. Alternatively, in the case of a gene mutation that results in loss of corneal transparency through loss of function of the encoded protein, the goal of genetic therapy would be to induce protein expression, either through replacement of the wild-type gene, activation of the gene promoter, or inhibition of a repressor of gene transcription.

Genetic Therapy for the TGBFI Dystrophies: A Work in Progress
While laser phototherapeutic keratectomy, lamellar and penetrating keratoplasty are effective means to address recurrent corneal erosions, visually significant subepithelial scarring or dystrophic deposits associated with the TGBFI dystrophies, each technique is associated with complications that are well known to all corneal surgeons. Recurrence following treatment is the norm rather than the exception, with the percentage of patients who developed a recurrence of dystrophic deposits following penetrating keratoplasty being approximately 43% for granular corneal dystrophy, 48–60% for lattice corneal dystrophy, and 88–100% for Reis-Bücklers and Thiel-Behnke corneal dystrophies [73–76]. While the median time to recurrence following penetrating keratoplasy in the published literature varies significantly, it is estimated to be as low as 2 years for the dystrophies of the Bowman layer [74]. The mean time to recurrence following phototherapeutic keratectomy has also been reported to be approximately 2 years in patients with Reis-Bücklers and Thiel-Behnke corneal dystrophies, and was even shorter (9.5 months) in patients who were homozygous for the mutant allele associated with granular corneal dystrophy, type 2 [76–81].

This need for repeated surgical intervention in a large percentage of patients with a TGBFI dystrophy has led to interest in nonsurgical means to prevent the development or recurrence of mutant TGFBIp production in the cornea. As the dystrophic deposits are localized to the corneas in affected patients, and are of a corneal as opposed to a blood-derived origin, only localized therapy is necessary [17, 82]. While TGBFIp is constitutively expressed by the human corneal epithelial cells, the amount that is produced by the epithelium and/or by the stromal keratocytes is increased significantly following injury or surgery via an increase in local *TGFB1* (MIM No. 190180) production, as has been reported following LASIK surgery [83–88]. RNA interference has been shown to effectively inhibit the TGFB1-induced increased expression of TGFBIp in human corneal epithelial cells [89] and to suppress expression of TGFBIp by 80% in an immortalized cell line [90]. However, the consequences of knocking down both the wild-type and the mutant TGBFIp in the cornea are not fully understood, and will only become clear once the physiologic significance of the role of TGFBIp in the cornea is further elucidated. It has been reported recently that Tgfbi$^{-/-}$ mice are prone to spontaneous tumor development, providing in vivo evidence to support findings from earlier in vitro studies that TGBFI functions as a tumor suppressor [91]. Therefore, animal models of the TGFBI dystrophies will need to be developed and therapeutic strategies such as RNA interference shown to be safe and effective before this or other genetic therapies for the corneal dystrophies progress to human trials.

References

1 Aldave AJ, Sonmez B: Elucidating the molecular genetic basis of the corneal dystrophies: are we there yet? Arch Ophthalmol 2007;125:177–186.

2 Weiss JS, Moller HU, Lisch W, et al: The IC3D classification of the corneal dystrophies. Cornea 2008; 27(suppl 2):S1–S83.

3 Hilton EN, Black GC, Manson FD, et al: De novo mutation in the BIGH3/TGFB1 gene causing granular corneal dystrophy. Br J Ophthalmol 2007;91: 1083–1084.

4 Zhao XC, Nakamura H, Subramanyam S, et al: Spontaneous and inheritable R555Q mutation in the TGFBI/BIGH3 gene in two unrelated families exhibiting Bowman's layer corneal dystrophy. Ophthalmology 2007;114:e39–e46.

5 Tanhehco TY, Eifrig DE Jr, Schwab IR, et al: Two cases of Reis-Bucklers corneal dystrophy (granular corneal dystrophy type III) caused by spontaneous mutations in the TGFBI gene. Arch Ophthalmol 2006;124:589–593.

6 Yellore VS, Sonmez B, Chen MC, et al: An unusual presentation of macular corneal dystrophy associated with uniparental isodisomy and a novel Leu173Pro mutation. Ophthalmic Genet 2007;28: 169–174.

7 Irvine AD, Corden LD, Swensson O, et al: Mutations in cornea-specific keratin K3 or K12 genes cause Meesmann's corneal dystrophy. Nat Genet 1997;16: 184–187.

8 Aldave AJ, Yellore VS, Vo RC, et al: Exclusion of positional candidate gene coding region mutations in the common posterior polymorphous corneal dystrophy 1 candidate gene interval. Cornea 2009; 28:801–807.

9 Aldave AJ, Yellore VS, Yu F, et al: Posterior polymorphous corneal dystrophy is associated with TCF8 gene mutations and abdominal hernia. Am J Med Genet A 2007;143A:2549–2556.

10 Heon E, Mathers WD, Alward WL, et al: Linkage of posterior polymorphous corneal dystrophy to 20q11. Hum Mol Genet 1995;4:485–488.

11 Krafchak CM, Pawar H, Moroi SE, et al: Mutations in TCF8 cause posterior polymorphous corneal dystrophy and ectopic expression of COL4A3 by corneal endothelial cells. Am J Hum Genet 2005; 77:694–708.

12 Liskova P, Tuft SJ, Gwilliam R, et al: Novel mutations in the ZEB1 gene identified in Czech and British patients with posterior polymorphous corneal dystrophy. Hum Mutat 2007;28:638.

13 Nguyen DQ, Hosseini M, Billingsley G, et al: Clinical phenotype of posterior polymorphous corneal dystrophy in a family with a novel ZEB1 mutation. Acta Ophthalmol 2010;88:695–699.

14 Biswas S, Munier FL, Yardley J, et al: Missense mutations in COL8A2, the gene encoding the alpha2 chain of type VIII collagen, cause two forms of corneal endothelial dystrophy. Hum Mol Genet 2001; 10:2415–2423.

15 Kobayashi A, Fujiki K, Murakami A, et al: Analysis of COL8A2 gene mutation in Japanese patients with Fuchs' endothelial dystrophy and posterior polymorphous dystrophy. Jpn J Ophthalmol 2004;48: 195–198.

16 Yellore VS, Rayner SA, Emmert-Buck L, et al: No pathogenic mutations identified in the COL8A2 gene or four positional candidate genes in patients with posterior polymorphous corneal dystrophy. Invest Ophthalmol Vis Sci 2005;46:1599–603.

17 El Kochairi I, Letovanec I, Uffer S, et al: Systemic investigation of keratoepithelin deposits in TGFBI/BIGH3-related corneal dystrophy. Mol Vis 2006;12: 461–466.

18 Lee JH, Chung SH, Stulting RD, et al: Effects of corneal neovascularization on the manifestations of Avellino corneal dystrophy (granular corneal dystrophy type II). Cornea 2006;25:914–918.

19 Klintworth GK, Oshima E, al-Rajhi A, et al: Macular corneal dystrophy in Saudi Arabia: a study of 56 cases and recognition of a new immunophenotype. Am J Ophthalmol 1997;124:9–18.

20 Bron AJ, Williams HP, Carruthers ME: Hereditary crystalline stromal dystrophy of Schnyder. 1. Clinical features of a family with hyperlipoproteinaemia. Br J Ophthalmol 1972;56:383–399.

21 Battisti C, Dotti MT, Malandrini A, et al: Schnyder corneal crystalline dystrophy: description of a new family with evidence of abnormal lipid storage in skin fibroblasts. Am J Med Genet 1998;75:35–39.

22 Aldave AJ, Rayner SA, King JA, et al: A unique corneal dystrophy of Bowman's layer and stroma associated with the Gly623Asp mutation in the transforming growth factor beta-induced (TGFBI) gene. Ophthalmology 2005;112:1017–1022.

23 Anderson NJ, Badawi DY, Grossniklaus HE, Stulting RD: Posterior polymorphous membranous dystrophy with overlapping features of iridocorneal endothelial syndrome. Arch Ophthalmol 2001;119: 624–625.

24 Stewart H, Black GC, Donnai D, et al: A mutation within exon 14 of the TGFBI (BIGH3) gene on chromosome 5q31 causes an asymmetric, late-onset form of lattice corneal dystrophy. Ophthalmology 1999;106:964–970.

25 Nakagawa Asahina S, Fujiki K, Enomoto Y, et al: Case of late onset and isolated lattice corneal dystrophy with Asn544Ser (N544S) mutation of transforming growth factor beta-induced (TGFBI, BIGH3) gene. Nippon Ganka Gakkai Zasshi 2004; 108:618–620.

26 Hirano K, Hotta Y, Nakamura M, et al: Late-onset form of lattice corneal dystrophy caused by leu527Arg mutation of the TGFBI gene. Cornea 2001;20:525–529.

27 Aldave AJ, Rayner SA, Kim BT, et al: Unilateral lattice corneal dystrophy associated with the novel His572del mutation in the TGFBI gene. Mol Vis 2006;12:142–146.

28 Aldave AJ: The clinical utility of genetic analysis in the diagnosis and management of inherited corneal disorders. Contemp Ophthalmol 2005;4:1–10.

29 Akhtar S, Meek KM, Ridgway AE, et al: Deposits and proteoglycan changes in primary and recurrent granular dystrophy of the cornea. Arch Ophthalmol 1999;117:310–321.

30 Johnson BL, Brown SI, Zaidman GW: A light and electron microscopic study of recurrent granular dystrophy of the cornea. Am J Ophthalmol 1981;92: 49–58.

31 Stone EM, Mathers WD, Rosenwasser GO, et al: Three autosomal dominant corneal dystrophies map to chromosome 5q. Nat Genet 1994;6:47–51.

32 Munier FL, Korvatska E, Djemai A, et al: Keratoepithelin mutations in four 5q31-linked corneal dystrophies. Nat Genet 1997;15:247–251.

33 Jiao X, Sultana A, Garg P, et al: Autosomal recessive corneal endothelial dystrophy (CHED2) is associated with mutations in SLC4A11. J Med Genet 2007; 44:64–68.

34 Sultana A, Garg P, Ramamurthy B, et al: Mutational spectrum of the SLC4A11 gene in autosomal recessive congenital hereditary endothelial dystrophy. Mol Vis 2007;13:1327–1332.

35 Kumar A, Bhattacharjee S, Prakash DR, Sadanand CS: Genetic analysis of two Indian families affected with congenital hereditary endothelial dystrophy: two novel mutations in SLC4A11. Mol Vis 2007;13: 39–46.

36 Aldave AJ, Yellore VS, Bourla N, et al: Autosomal recessive CHED associated with novel compound heterozygous mutations in SLC4A11. Cornea 2007; 26:896–900.

37 Ramprasad VL, Ebenezer ND, Aung T, et al: Novel SLC4A11 mutations in patients with recessive congenital hereditary endothelial dystrophy (CHED2). Hum Mut 2007;28:522–523.

38 Vithana EN, Morgan P, Sundaresan P, et al: Mutations in sodium-borate cotransporter SLC4A11 cause recessive congenital hereditary endothelial dystrophy (CHED2). Nat Genet 2006;38:755–757.

39 Hemadevi B, Veitia RA, Srinivasan M, et al: Identification of mutations in the SLC4A11 gene in patients with recessive congenital hereditary endothelial dystrophy. Arch Ophthalmol 2008;126: 700–708.

40 Aldahmesh MA, Khan AO, Meyer BF, Alkuraya FS: Mutational spectrum of SLC4A11 in autosomal recessive CHED in Saudi Arabia. Invest Ophthalmol Vis Sci 2009;50:4142–4145.

41 Shah SS, Al-Rajhi A, Brandt JD, et al: Mutation in the SLC4A11 gene associated with autosomal recessive congenital hereditary endothelial dystrophy in a large Saudi family. Ophthalmic Genet 2008;29:41–45.
42 Li S, Tiab L, Jiao X, et al: Mutations in PIP5K3 are associated with François-Neetens mouchetée fleck corneal dystrophy. Am J Hum Genet 2005;77: 54–63.
43 Aldave AJ, Rayner SA, Salem AK, et al: No pathogenic mutations identified in the COL8A1 and COL8A2 genes in familial Fuchs corneal dystrophy. Invest Ophthalmol Vis Sci 2006;47:3787–3790.
44 Aldave AJ, Yellore VS, Principe AH, et al: Candidate gene screening for posterior polymorphous dystrophy. Cornea 2005;24:151–155.
45 Gwilliam R, Liskova P, Filipec M, et al: Posterior polymorphous corneal dystrophy in Czech families maps to chromosome 20 and excludes the VSX1 gene. Invest Ophthalmol Vis Sci 2005;46:4480–4484.
46 Yellore VS, Khan MA, Bourla N, et al: Identification of mutations in UBIAD1 following exclusion of coding mutations in the chromosome 1p36 locus for Schnyder crystalline corneal dystrophy. Mol Vis 2007;13:1777–1782.
47 Germain DP: Pseudoxanthoma elasticum: evidence for the existence of a pseudogene highly homologous to the ABCC6 gene. J Med Genet 2001;38: 457–461.
48 North KN, Yang N, Wattanasirichaigoon D, et al: A common nonsense mutation results in alpha-actinin-3 deficiency in the general population. Nat Genet 1999;21:353–354.
49 Zhang X, Yeung KY, Pang CP, Fu W: Mutation analysis of retinitis pigmentosa 1 gene in Chinese with retinitis pigmentosa. Zhonghua Yi Xue Yi Chuan Xue Za Zhi 2002;19:194–197.
50 Heon E, Greenberg A, Kopp KK, et al: VSX1: a gene for posterior polymorphous dystrophy and keratoconus. Hum Mol Genet 2002;11:1029–1036.
51 Mintz-Hittner HA, Semina EV, Frishman LJ, et al: VSX1 (RINX) mutation with craniofacial anomalies, empty sella, corneal endothelial changes, and abnormal retinal and auditory bipolar cells. Ophthalmology 2004;111:828–836.
52 Valleix S, Nedelec B, Rigaudiere F, et al: H244R VSX1 is associated with selective cone ON bipolar cell dysfunction and macular degeneration in a PPCD family. Invest Ophthalmol Vis Sci 2006;47: 48–54.
53 Gottsch JD, Sundin OH, Liu SH, et al: Inheritance of a novel COL8A2 mutation defines a distinct early-onset subtype of fuchs corneal dystrophy. Invest Ophthalmol Vis Sci 2005;46:1934–1939.
54 Liskova P, Prescott Q, Bhattacharya SS, Tuft SJ: British family with early-onset Fuchs' endothelial corneal dystrophy associated with p.L450W mutation in the COL8A2 gene. Br J Ophthalmol 2007;91: 1717–1718.
55 Vithana EN, Morgan PE, Ramprasad V, et al: SLC4A11 mutations in Fuchs endothelial corneal dystrophy. Hum Mol Genet 2008;17:656–666.
56 Klintworth GK, Vogel FS: Macular corneal dystrophy. An inherited acid mucopolysaccharide storage disease of the corneal fibroblast. Am J Pathol 1964; 45:565–586.
57 Hassell JR, Newsome DA, Krachmer JH, Rodrigues MM: Macular corneal dystrophy: failure to synthesize a mature keratan sulfate proteoglycan. Proc Natl Acad Sci USA 1980;77:3705–3709.
58 Midura RJ, Hascall VC, MacCallum DK, et al: Proteoglycan biosynthesis by human corneas from patients with types 1 and 2 macular corneal dystrophy. J Biol Chem 1990;265:15947–15955.
59 Akama TO, Nishida K, Nakayama J, et al: Macular corneal dystrophy type I and type II are caused by distinct mutations in a new sulphotransferase gene. Nat Genet 2000;26:237–241.
60 Bonanno JA: Identity and regulation of ion transport mechanisms in the corneal endothelium. Prog Retin Eye Res 2003;22:69–94.
61 Thapa N, Lee BH, Kim IS: TGFBIp/betaig-h3 protein: a versatile matrix molecule induced by TGF-beta. Int J Biochem Cell Biol 2007;39:2183–2194.
62 Lopez IA, Rosenblatt MI, Kim C, et al: Slc4a11 gene disruption in mice: cellular targets of sensorineuronal abnormalities. J Biol Chem 2009;284: 26882–26896.
63 Schmitt-Bernard CF, Chavanieu A, Herrada G, et al: BIGH3 (TGFBI) Arg124 mutations influence the amyloid conversion of related peptides in vitro. Eur J Biochem 2002;269:5149–5156.
64 Bainbridge JW, Smith AJ, Barker SS, et al: Effect of gene therapy on visual function in Leber's congenital amaurosis. N Engl J Med 2008;358:2231–2239.
65 Cideciyan AV, Hauswirth WW, Aleman TS, et al: Human RPE65 gene therapy for Leber congenital amaurosis: persistence of early visual improvements and safety at 1 year. Hum Gene Ther 2009;20: 999–1004.
66 Mancuso K, Hauswirth WW, Li Q, et al: Gene therapy for red-green colour blindness in adult primates. Nature 2009;461:784–787.
67 Klausner EA, Peer D, Chapman RL, et al: Corneal gene therapy. J Control Release 2007;124: 107–133.
68 Mohan RR, Sharma A, Netto MV, et al: Gene therapy in the cornea. Prog Retin Eye Res 2005;24: 537–559.

69 Borras T, Gabelt BT, Klintworth GK, et al: Noninvasive observation of repeated adenoviral GFP gene delivery to the anterior segment of the monkey eye in vivo. J Gene Med 2001;3:437–449.
70 Klebe S, Sykes PJ, Coster DJ, et al: Prolongation of sheep corneal allograft survival by ex vivo transfer of the gene encoding interleukin-10. Transplantation 2001;71:1214–1220.
71 Bennett J, Maguire AM: Gene therapy for ocular disease. Mol Ther 2000;1:501–505.
72 Pleyer U, Dannowski H: Delivery of genes via liposomes to corneal endothelial cells. Drug News Perspect 2002;15:283–289.
73 Lyons CJ, McCartney AC, Kirkness CM, et al: Granular corneal dystrophy. Visual results and pattern of recurrence after lamellar or penetrating keratoplasty. Ophthalmology 1994;101:1812–1817.
74 Marcon AS, Cohen EJ, Rapuano CJ, Laibson PR: Recurrence of corneal stromal dystrophies after penetrating keratoplasty. Cornea 2003;22:19–21.
75 Meisler DM, Fine M: Recurrence of the clinical signs of lattice corneal dystrophy (type I) in corneal transplants. Am J Ophthalmol 1984;97:210–214.
76 Sorour HM, Yee SB, Peterson NJ, et al: Recurrence of chromosome 10 Thiel-Behnke corneal dystrophy (CDB2) after excimer laser phototherapeutic keratectomy or penetrating keratoplasty. Cornea 2005; 24:45–50.
77 Dinh R, Rapuano CJ, Cohen EJ, Laibson PR: Recurrence of corneal dystrophy after excimer laser phototherapeutic keratectomy. Ophthalmology 1999;106:1490–1497.
78 Dogru M, Katakami C, Nishida T, Yamanaka A: Alteration of the ocular surface with recurrence of granular/avellino corneal dystrophy after phototherapeutic keratectomy: report of five cases and literature review. Ophthalmology 2001;108: 810–817.
79 Ellies P, Bejjani RA, Bourges JL, et al: Phototherapeutic keratectomy for BIGH3-linked corneal dystrophy recurring after penetrating keratoplasty. Ophthalmology 2003;110:1119–1125.
80 Inoue T, Watanabe H, Yamamoto S, et al: Recurrence of corneal dystrophy resulting from an R124H Big-h3 mutation after phototherapeutic keratectomy. Cornea 2002;21:570–573.
81 Orndahl MJ, Fagerholm PP: Treatment of corneal dystrophies with phototherapeutic keratectomy. J Refract Surg 1998;14:129–135.
82 Karring H, Valnickova Z, Thogersen IB, et al: Evidence against a blood derived origin for transforming growth factor beta induced protein in corneal disorders caused by mutations in the TGFBI gene. Mol Vis 2007;13:997–1004.
83 Aldave AJ, Sonmez B, Forstot SL, et al: A clinical and histopathologic examination of accelerated TGFBIp deposition after LASIK in combined granular-lattice corneal dystrophy. Am J Ophthalmol 2007;143:416–419.
84 Banning CS, Kim WC, Randleman JB, et al: Exacerbation of Avellino corneal dystrophy after LASIK in North America. Cornea 2006;25: 482–484.
85 Jun RM, Tchah H, Kim TI, et al: Avellino corneal dystrophy after LASIK. Ophthalmology 2004;111: 463–468.
86 Kim TI, Kim T, Kim SW, Kim EK: Comparison of corneal deposits after LASIK and PRK in eyes with granular corneal dystrophy type II. J Refract Surg 2008;24:392–395.
87 Kim TI, Roh MI, Grossniklaus HE, et al: Deposits of transforming growth factor-beta-induced protein in granular corneal dystrophy type II after LASIK. Cornea 2008;27:28–32.
88 Wan XH, Lee HC, Stulting RD, et al: Exacerbation of Avellino corneal dystrophy after laser in situ keratomileusis. Cornea 2002;21:223–226.
89 Yellore VS, Rayner SA, Aldave AJ: TGFB1-induced extracellular expression of TGFBIp and inhibition of TGFBIp expression by RNA interference in a human corneal epithelial cell line. Invest Ophthalmol Vis Sci 2011;52:757–763.
90 Yuan C, Zins EJ, Clark AF, Huang AJ: Suppression of keratoepithelin and myocilin by small interfering RNAs (siRNA) in vitro. Mol Vis 2007;13: 2083–2095.
91 Zhang Y, Wen G, Shao G, et al: TGFBI deficiency predisposes mice to spontaneous tumor development. Cancer Res 2009;69:37–44.

Dr. Anthony J. Aldave
The Jules Stein Eye Institute
100 Stein Plaza, UCLA
Los Angeles, CA 90095 (USA)
Tel. +1 310 206 7202, E-Mail aldave@jsei.ucla.edu

Lisch W, Seitz B (eds): Corneal Dystrophies.
Dev Ophthalmol. Basel, Karger, 2011, vol 48, pp 67–96

Differential Diagnosis of Schnyder Corneal Dystrophy

Jayne S. Weiss[a] · Arbi J. Khemichian[b]

[a]Department of Ophthalmology, Louisiana State University Health Science Center, New Orleans, La.;
[b]Kresge Eye Institute, Wayne State University School of Medicine, Detroit, Mich., USA

Abstract

Schnyder corneal dystrophy (SCD) is a rare corneal dystrophy characterized by abnormally increased deposition of cholesterol and phospholipids in the cornea leading to progressive vision loss. SCD is inherited as an autosomal dominant trait with high penetrance and has been mapped to the *UBIAD1* gene on chromosome 1p36.3. Although 2/3 of SCD patients also have systemic hypercholesterolemia, the incidence of hypercholesterolemia is also increased in unaffected members of SCD pedigrees. Consequently, SCD is thought to result from a local metabolic defect in the cornea. The corneal findings in SCD are very predictable depending on the age of the individual, with initial central corneal haze and/or crystals, subsequent appearance of arcus lipoides in the third decade and formation of midperipheral haze in the late fourth decade. Because only 50% of affected patients have corneal crystals, the International Committee for Classification of Corneal Dystrophies recently changed the original name of this dystrophy from Schnyder crystalline corneal dystrophy to Schnyder corneal dystrophy. Diagnosis of affected individuals without crystalline deposits is often delayed and these individuals are frequently misdiagnosed. The differential diagnosis of the SCD patient includes other diseases with crystalline deposits such as cystinosis, tyrosinemia, Bietti crystalline dystrophy, hyperuricemia/gout, multiple myeloma, monoclonal gammopathy, infectious crystalline keratopathy, and Dieffenbachia keratitis. Depositions from drugs such as gold in chrysiasis, chlorpromazine, chloroquine, and clofazamine can also result in corneal deposits and are different from SCD. Diseases of systemic lipid metabolism that cause corneal opacification, such as lecithin-cholesterol acyltransferase deficiency, fish eye disease and Tangier disease, should also be considered although these are autosomal recessive disorders.

Schnyder Corneal Dystrophy

Definition

Schnyder corneal dystrophy (SCD) is a rare dystrophy characterized by abnormally increased deposition of cholesterol and phospholipids in the cornea leading to progressive vision loss.

Genetics
SCD is inherited as an autosomal dominant trait with high penetrance and has been mapped to the *UBIAD1* gene [1, 2, 3] on chromosome 1p36.3 [4].

Pathophysiology
The exact pathogenesis of SCD remains unknown. *UBIAD1* gene has been shown to code for prenyltransferase proteins which have a role in the direct and indirect control of intracellular cholesterol storage and transport [2, 3]. This is postulated to result in a localized defect of lipid metabolism. It has been demonstrated in affected versus normal corneas that the cholesterol content increases 10-fold and the phospholipid content increases 5-fold [5]. Immunohistochemical analysis has revealed the preferential deposition of apolipoprotein components of high-density lipoprotein (HDL), but not of low-density lipoprotein (LDL) [5]. This finding suggests an abnormal metabolism of HDL in the cornea with SCD.

Prevalence
SCD is considered rare and there are less than 150 articles in the published literature [6].

Systemic Findings
The major systemic finding in SCD is hypercholesterolemia. Elevated cholesterol levels have been shown to be present in two thirds of patients with SCD and in unaffected members of SCD pedigrees [7, 8]. However, the severity of dyslipidemia does not directly correlate with the amount of corneal lipid deposition [9]. Also, long-term follow-up studies have determined that lowering of systemic cholesterol does not prevent progression of the corneal disease [10]. In fact, patients affected by the corneal dystrophy may have normal serum lipid, lipoprotein, or cholesterol levels [11, 12], while unaffected family members of these SCD pedigrees may have elevated levels.

Although rare, the presence of genu valgum, a condition where the knees angle in and touch one another when the legs are straightened, has also been shown to be associated with SCD [13, 14].

Ocular Findings
While SCD has been diagnosed as early as at 17 months of age in patients with crowded needle-shaped corneal crystals, diagnosing SCD is often more challenging in affected individuals without crystals and may be delayed to the fourth decade. Crystalline deposition is only found in approximately 50% of SCD patients (fig. 1) [15]. While many authors continue to believe that the presence of crystals is integral to the diagnosis of SCD, this is incorrect. In fact, corneal biopsy has been reported in patients with classical findings of SCD without crystals [16]. However, the diagnosis should be able to made solely on clinical exam. Subjectively, patients usually complain of glare and loss of photopic vision as the corneal haze progresses. Scotopic

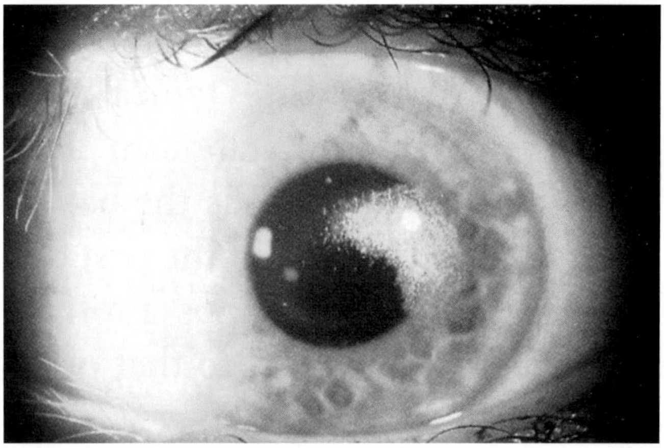

Fig. 1. Early subepithelial deposits of crystals in an arc formation in a young individual with SCD. Courtesy of Jayne Weiss.

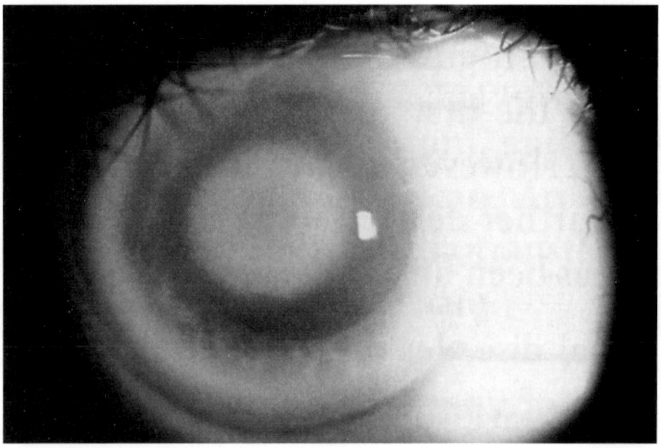

Fig. 2. Mid aged individual with SCD and central corneal disciform opacity, mid-peripheral haze and arcus lipoides. Courtesy of Jayne Weiss.

vision usually decreases minimally associated with the progression of corneal opacification. An 18-year study showed that the mean Snellen uncorrected visual acuity was between 20/25 and 20/30 in patients younger than 40 years and between 20/30 and 20/40 in patients aged 40 years or older [6]. Progressive loss of corneal sensation has also been found to be more profound in advanced cases. Confocal biomicroscopy has revealed absence of corneal nerves and deposition of large extracellular crystals and reflective matrix resulting in disruption of basal epithelial and subepithelial nerve plexus [16]. In those patients younger than 24 years of age, only a central panstromal opacity and/or subepithelial crystalline deposition is noted. Patients aged 23–38 years nearly all have an arcus lipoides (fig. 2) and acuity may be diminished if measured under daylight conditions. Corneal sensation also begins to decrease in this age range. In patients 39 years and older, a midperipheral, panstromal corneal haze appears that

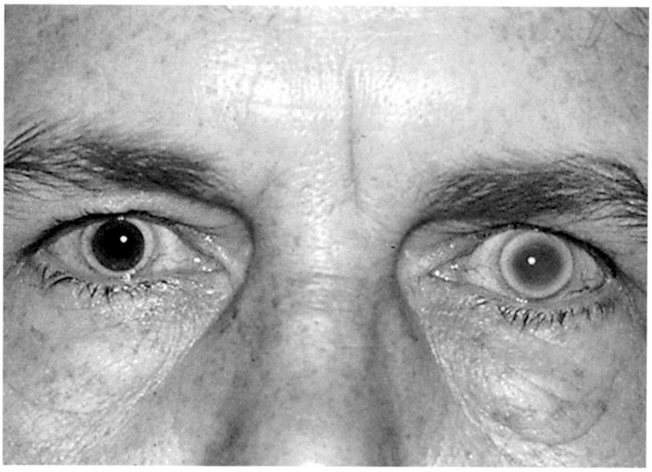

Fig. 3. Elderly woman with SCD and difuse corneal haze and prominent arcus lipoides in the left eye. The right eye has had prior penetrating keratoplasty so that the central donor cornea is clear while arcus lipoides causes haziness of the peripheral host cornea. Courtesy of Jayne Weiss.

fills in the area between the central opacity and the peripheral arcus (fig. 3). Often, the arcus is dense enough to be seen without a slit lamp.

The subepithelial location of crystalline deposits on ocular coherence tomography examination extends from the basal epithelium layer to a depth of 80–150 μm [17]. When viewed with electron microscopy, there are unesterified and esterified cholesterol particles in the basal epithelium and Bowman layer [18].

Treatment

Although slowly progressive and moderately debilitating visually, the 18-year follow-up of SCD patients revealed that 54% of patients with SCD aged 50 years and older and 77% of patients aged 70 years and older had corneal transplant surgery [penetrating keratoplasty (PKP)] [6]. The visual acuity of these patients preoperatively ranged from 20/25 to 20/400 suggesting that even though excellent scotopic vision continues until middle age, most patients had PKP by the seventh decade due to progressive corneal opacification, which may result in glare and disproportionate loss of photopic vision. Systemically, there was no evidence of increased mortality from cardiovascular disease in SCD [6].

Lecithin-Cholesterol Acyltransferase Deficiency and Fish Eye Disease

Definition

Lecithin-cholesterol acyltransferase (LCAT) deficiency and fish eye disease (FED) are both entities that result from deficiency of the LCAT enzyme [19]. LCAT deficiency is defined by deficient LCAT activity towards HDL and LDL and was first reported in 1967 in a Norwegian family [20]. FED is defined by decreased LCAT activity against HDL only and was initially described in 2 families of Swedish origin [21]. Residual LCAT activity is still detectable in FED.

Genetics

Both familial LCAT deficiency and FED are autosomal recessive disorders caused by mutations of the *LCAT* gene [22] mapped to chromosome 16q22 [23]. The distinct mutation type determines whether the result is LCAT deficiency or FED [24].

Pathophysiology

LCAT plays an important role in lipoprotein metabolism. The enzyme is synthesized in the liver and circulates in blood plasma as a complex with components of HDL. Cholesterol from peripheral cells is transferred to HDL particles, esterified through the action of LCAT on HDL, and incorporated into the core of the lipoprotein. The cholesterol ester is thereby transported to the liver [19]. A lack of LCAT activity leads to excess accumulation of free (unesterified) cholesterol in tissues such as the cornea and kidney.

Prevalence

Both familial LCAT deficiency and FED are rare. As of 2005, there were about 50 described cases of LCAT deficiency and an unknown number of cases with FED [25]. There are no reliable figures as to the true prevalence for each disease. One article showed one of the highest prevalences of LCAT deficiency to be in a secluded area of Norway, where 4% of the population was found to have the heterozygous mutation of the LCAT enzyme [26].

Systemic Findings

The most common systemic findings in LCAT deficiency are normocytic anemia, corneal opacities, renal insufficiency, and rarely atherosclerosis. One report showed that 92% of patients were found to be anemic and 76% had proteinuria at diagnosis [27]. In contrast, the only significant finding in FED is corneal opacities [28, 29].

Basic laboratory tests such as a complete blood count, complete metabolic panel for kidney function and lipid profile can differentiate the 2 rare diseases. In familial LCAT deficiency, the plasma may show a 5-fold increase in levels of unesterified cholesterol, very-low-density lipoprotein and triglycerides. The levels of LDL are found to be normal, while those of esterified cholesterol and HDL are reduced by up to 90%. Levels of HDL are usually less than 10 mg/dl [30]. This increase in free cholesterol may result in turbidity of plasma [31, 32]. Although FED shows a similar lipid profile to LCAT deficiency, the main distinction is the near-normal ratio of unesterified to total cholesterol in plasma. This normal ratio is due to residual activity of the gene in FED. In fact, heterozygotes can nearly show half the normal amount of LCAT activity [33].

Regarding renal disease, severe cases of LCAT deficiency may eventually lead to renal function deterioration with eventual need for dialysis and/or renal transplantation [30]. There is no renal pathology seen with FED. Other findings in severe disease include hypertension, atherosclerosis and xanthelasma.

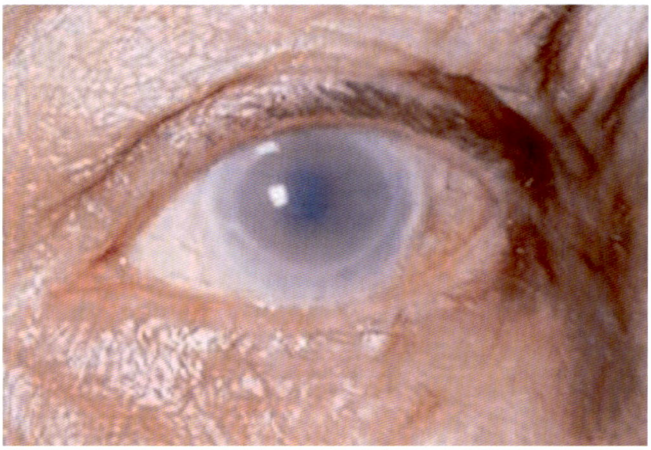

Fig. 4. Corneal opacification with peripheral ring opacity in patient with Lecithin Cholesterol Acyltransferase Deficiency. Courtesy of Walter Lisch.

Ocular Findings

Ocular findings in LCAT deficiency usually present in the third to fourth decade of life, while those of FED can be seen as early as prior to age 20 [34, 35]. The overall opacity pattern of LCAT deficiency is the same in all cases and is pathognomic for the disease: a diffuse cloudiness composed of innumerable minute grayish dots and ringlike condensation in the periphery, only resembling an arcus lipoides [27] (fig. 4). However, this ring differs from typical arcus lipoides in its indistinct peripheral margin and a limbal zone of mild opacities containing vacuoles. The diffuse cloudiness can have a shagreenlike appearance and should be differentiated from the classic crocodile shagreen. The peripheral ring represents a landmark of LCAT deficiency and FED [27]. These dot opacifications are not crystalline and do not impair visual acuity. Secondary amyloidosis of the cornea has also been reported [31]. The main subjective findings are complaints of glare disability and photophobia [27].

Ocular findings in FED are more pronounced but identical to those of LCAT deficiency. With progression, the cornea may show diffuse opacification with phospholipid and cholesterol having been observed in all corneal layers and lead to significant vision loss as early as at 15 years of age [30]. This appearance is similar to the eyes of a boiled fish, which is how the name of the disease was created.

Lecithin-Cholesterol Acyltransferase Deficiency and Fish Eye Disease versus Schnyder Corneal Dystrophy

When comparing LCAT deficiency and FED to SCD, there are numerous differences to help distinguish all 3 entities. Both LCAT deficiency and FED are inherited in an autosomal recessive manner while SCD has autosomal dominant inheritance. Systemically, SCD has a normal level of LCAT enzyme activity. Both LCAT deficiency and FED show abnormally low levels of HDL, usually below 10 mg/dl, and normal LDL levels, while SCD shows normal HDL levels with possibly elevated levels of LDL and esterified cholesterol [36]. SCD is often associated with a true arcus lipoides. LCAT deficiency and FED represent a peripheral ringlike opacification which is completely different to a true arcus lipoides. The noncrystalline type of SCD with a facultative arcus lipoides is to be distinguished from LCAT deficiency and FED. Neither LCAT deficiency nor FED has crystalline deposits in the cornea. In LCAT deficiency, the abnormal corneal dots are more prominent peripherally and occur in all layers of the stroma [37]. FED does not exhibit any crystals or dot deposition. In SCD, approximately 50% of patients have crystalline deposits that are more prominent centrally and paracentrally and occur in the subepithelial layer [6].

Treatment

Whole blood or plasma transfusion has been tried to replace the LCAT enzyme in some patients with familial LCAT deficiency, but this did not correct anemia, proteinuria, or lipoprotein abnormalities [38]. Also, renal replacement therapy by dialysis is necessary in those individuals who develop kidney failure. Although not reported yet in the literature, LCAT gene therapy or liver transplantation may eventually be potential treatments that could address the underlying genetic defect. Although rare, PKP has been reported for severe corneal opacification. One patient with FED who had undergone PKP and had a 2-year follow-up was found to have a clear graft. The final distance vision of the surgical eye was 20/25 [39]. Meanwhile, another study described a patient with LCAT deficiency who had prolonged wound healing after PKP. The epithelial wound did not close until the 32nd postoperative day [31].

Tangier Disease

Definition

Tangier disease is a systemic disease characterized by markedly reduced levels of plasma HDL resulting in accumulation of cholesterol-rich lipids such as cholesterol esters [40] in different tissues.

Genetics

Tangier disease is inherited in an autosomal recessive mode and results from mutations in the ATP-binding cassette transporter *(ABCA1)* gene [41] on chromosome 9q31.

Pathophysiology

Genetic mutation in the *ABCA1* gene results in abnormalities of the cholesterol efflux regulatory protein, which plays a central role in intracellular cholesterol transport [42]. This inability to transport cholesterol out of cells leads to a deficiency of HDL in the circulation and causes buildup of cholesterol in cells. Severity of HDL deficiency varies with genetic status with 50% reduction in heterozygotes and a nearly complete decrease in homozygotes. This buildup of cholesterol can lead to cell toxicity and death [43].

Prevalence
Tangier disease is rare and there are no reported studies on its prevalence.

Systemic Findings
Prior publications review systemic findings in Tangier patients from 2 to 67 years of age [44]. Findings include enlarged yellow-orange tonsils, liver, spleen and lymph nodes as well as peripheral neuropathy. Electrophysiologic studies demonstrated neuropathy to be predominantly due to axonal sensorimotor polyneuropathy with signs of chronic denervation from deposition of fat droplets in axons and Schwann cells [45]. Although not to the degree of patients with familial hypercholesterolemia, Tangier patients do show an increased risk of premature vascular disease [46, 47]. Laboratory studies show severely reduced serum HDL (<5 mg/dl), decreased total cholesterol and apolipoprotein A-I, and elevated levels of triglycerides [44, 45, 47].

Ocular Findings
Patients with Tangier disease may have cicatricial ectropion and slowly progressive corneal clouding with granular stromal haze [48]. Studies with slit lamp biomicroscopy and confocal microscopy have demonstrated bilateral corneal opacification results from abnormal corneal lipid deposition. There is no arcus lipoides or corneal crystalline deposition. The corneal clouding may minimally reduce vision to the range of 20/25 to 20/40. However, marked visual decrease can result if ectropion and incomplete eyelid closure lead to exposure keratopathy and corneal scarring [48]. If conjunctival biopsy is performed, histopathology demonstrates birefringent lipid particles that are predominantly present in degenerating pericytes of the conjunctival vessels [49].

Tangier Disease versus Schnyder Corneal Dystrophy
Although Tangier disease and SCD both have abnormal corneal deposition, there are many differences between the 2 diseases. Tangier disease is inherited in an autosomal recessive mode while SCD is inherited in an autosomal dominant mode. In Tangier disease, there is marked reduction in systemic HDL, while SCD patients have normal HDL levels. SCD patients aged 23 years and older frequently demonstrate an arcus lipoides while this finding is not present in Tangier disease. While approximately 50% of SCD patients have corneal crystalline deposits, corneal crystals are not found in Tangier disease. The corneal clouding in SCD is limited to the central and midperipheral cornea whereas that of Tangier disease may be seen diffusely.

Treatment
There is no specific treatment for Tangier disease. The treatment of decreased HDL with medication is usually ineffective. Organs such as the spleen and tonsils must be removed if there is extensive accumulation of cholesterol. Arteriosclerosis may be treated through angioplasty or bypass surgery [34].

Cystinosis

Definition

Cystinosis is an inherited lysosomal storage disorder characterized by abnormal deposition of intralysosomal cystine [50]. A cellular metabolic disorder of transport across the lysosomal membrane results in membrane-bound collection of cystine and acid phosphatase [51]. This defect of lysosomal cystine efflux causes 3 separate clinical forms of the disease: infantile nephropathic, juvenile and ocular nonnephropathic [52].

Genetics

Cystinosis is inherited in an autosomal recessive mode and results from mutations in the cystinosin gene *(CTNS)* located on chromosome 17p13. The gene, *CTNS,* codes for the lysosomal membrane protein called cystinosin and functions in exporting cystine from lysosyme [53]. At least 55 such mutations have been described in patients with cystinosis, with the clinical phenotype segregating with specific defects. For example, mild mutations in the *CTNS* gene still allow residual mRNA production with continued lysosomal cystine transport, which results in lower levels of cellular cystine and less severe clinical findings than those in nephropathic cystinosis [52]. By far the most common mutation is a 57,257-bp deletion of Northern European origin encompassing most of the *CTNS* gene [54].

Pathophysiology

Normally, ingested protein enters the lysosome where it is broken down to its component amino acids, including cysteine, by acid hydrolases. Cysteine may then be broken down further to cystine. In individuals with normal gene function, both cystine and cysteine can then enter the cytoplasm from the lysosomes where they are incorporated into protein or degraded to inorganic sulfate for excretion. In cystinosis, a defect in cystinosin prevents cystine from entering the cytoplasm and it remains trapped in lysosomes. The abnormal accumulation of cystine deposits as birefringent, hexagonal, or rectangular crystals within cells.

Prevalence

The incidence of congenital cystinosis has been estimated as 1 in 100,000 to 1 in 200,000, although this varies depending on geography [55].

Systemic Findings

Infantile nephropathic cystinosis results from abnormal cystine accumulation [33] causing decreased reabsorption of electrolytes and nutrients. Proximal tubular function is damaged because of this excess accumulation of cystine. Ninety-five percent of infants between 6 and 12 months of age are reported to have Fanconi syndrome and develop chronic renal failure by age 8–12 [57]. Severe kidney problems may lead to the loss of important minerals, salts, fluids, and other nutrients. This loss of nutrients not only impairs growth, but may also result in soft bowed bones, especially in the legs. The nutrient imbalances in the body lead to increased urination, thirst, dehydration, and abnormally acidic blood.

Hypothyroidism occurs in 50% of cases and is seen by age 5–10. Other systemic findings include myopathy, which may be seen in 20% of patients aged 12–40 and can present as difficulty swallowing. About 10–15% of patients have diabetes mellitus, 5% of males have hypogonadism, 70% show pulmonary dysfunction, and nearly 100% show central nervous system calcifications between ages 21 and 40 years [57]. Unless treated by renal transplant, infantile nephropathic cystinosis is fatal within the first decade of life.

Adolescent nephropathic cystinosis initially manifests itself around the age of 10–12 years. Clinically the disorder shows a slowly progressive glomerular insufficiency with proteinuria as the main finding rather than tubular damage that occurs in infantile cystinosis. There is no excess aminoaciduria and stature is normal.

In the adult form, also known as ocular nonnephropathic cystinosis, patients only present with ocular findings. There are no renal or other systemic findings.

Ocular Findings

Most patients with cystinosis complain of photophobia. One study found significantly lower contrast sensitivities in patients with cystinosis compared to normals, which may be caused by corneal and retinal crystalline deposition [58]. On slit lamp exam, ocular findings in cystinosis include the deposition of fine punctiform and polychromatic cystine crystals in the conjunctiva, corneal stroma, trabecular meshwork and peripheral retina. The densest concentration of these anterior stromal crystals occurs in the peripheral cornea although they may also occur centrally [59].

In a large study of 170 patients with congenital nephropathic cystinosis, infants in the first year of life had absent or minimal corneal crystals, but by 16 months of age, nearly all patients had visible crystals. Corneal deposition plateaued by early adolescence [60]. In contrast, the earliest finding of crystals in patients with nonnephropathic cystinosis has been reported to be in the mid-teen years [61]. This group also has approximately 50% less crystals than patients of the same age who have nephropathic disease [60]. The most common posterior segment finding is retinal pigment epithelial mottling, which can manifest in early infancy. This may lead to visual field constriction and ERG rod and cone response reduction in older patients [62].

Ancillary imaging modalities have been used to facilitate diagnosis. In one study of patients with nephropathic cystinosis, in vitro confocal microscopy and anterior segment optical coherence tomography demonstrated corneal crystals that appeared as hyperreflective punctate deposits, concentrated within the anterior stroma. Measured with anterior segment optical coherence tomography, the mean depth of crystal deposition in the central cornea was found to be 291.4 μm (range, 200–

531 μm) with a mean corneal thickness of 543 μm [59]. There were no crystals deposited on the endothelium. Crystals measured 1–175 μm in length and 1–30 μm in thickness.

Cystinosis versus Schnyder Corneal Dystrophy

Although both cystinosis and SCD may manifest corneal crystalline deposits, there are many ways to differentiate the 2 diseases. The pattern of inheritance is autosomal recessive in cystinosis while autosomal dominant in SCD. Systemic findings such as severe kidney disease and thyroid dysfunction occur in congenital and adolescent forms of cystinosis but do not occur in SCD. Hypercholesterolemia occurs in the 66% of SCD patients, but is not a characteristic finding in individuals with cystinosis [6]. Ocular findings may be differentiated based on location of crystal deposition in the cornea and other ocular structures. Solitary punctiform crystals in cystinosis occur throughout all layers of the cornea except the endothelium while crowded needle-shaped crystals in SCD occur in the anterior stroma. In addition, crystals in cystinosis are more prominent peripherally while in SCD they are more prominent centrally and paracentrally. The deposition of cystine crystals within retinal pigment epithelial cells and trabecular meshwork are also features unique to cystinosis that are not found in SCD.

Treatment

Prior treatment of cystinosis was limited to treating metabolic acidosis and replacing electrolytes lost in the urine. Today cysteamine and renal transplantation has improved quality of life especially in nephropathic disease. Recent studies have shown that if diagnosis is established early and cysteamine therapy is started before symptoms develop, the prognosis for glomerular function is especially good and patients may live into their third decade [57]. Cysteamine has even been shown to improve other systemic problems by obviating the need for levothyroxine therapy in patients with thyroid disease [63]. The effect of cysteamine on ocular tissue has also been noted. Topical cysteamine decreases the number of corneal crystals in treated eyes within 4–5 months, if patients begin therapy before 2 years of age [64]. Corneal cystine crystals dissolved with topical 0.55% cysteamine drops, between 6 and 12 times per day in 10 patients of different ages with nephropathic cystinosis, within 8–41 months. Early institution of oral cysteamine treatment is also shown to limit visual loss and decrease posterior segment complications [65].

Tyrosinemia Type II (Richner-Hanhart Syndrome)

Definition

Tyrosinemia type II, otherwise know as Richner-Hanhart syndrome or oculocutaneous tyrosinemia, is a disorder of tyrosine metabolism due to the deficiency of the cytosolic fraction of hepatic tyrosine aminotransferase [66]. Richner in 1938 and Hanhart in 1947 described this clinical syndrome independently [67].

Genetics

Tyrosinemia type II is an autosomal recessive disease which results from a mutation in the tyrosine aminotransferase gene *(TAT)* located on chromosome 16q22.1–q22.3.

Pathophysiology

The *TAT* gene is responsible for coding for TAT protein. In tyrosinemia, mutations in the *TAT* gene result in deficiency of hepatic TAT enzyme, the rate-limiting enzyme of tyrosine catabolism. TAT is the first in a series of 5 enzymes that converts tyrosine to smaller molecules, which are excreted by the kidneys or used in reactions that produce energy. When there is insufficient TAT, excess tyrosine deposits in tissues and is excreted through the urinary system resulting in tyrosinuria with increases in urinary phenolic acids, N-acetyl tyrosine, and tyramine. The metabolism of other amino acids and renal and hepatic function are otherwise normal [68].

Prevalence

Although the exact prevalence of tyrosinemia type II is unknown, it is considered a rare disease, which is defined by the National Institutes of Health as occurring in less than 1 in 250,000 individuals.

Systemic Findings

The threshold levels of tyrosine for appearance of clinical manifestation is reported as 1,000 μmol/l. Skin manifestations usually begin after the first year of life, but may occur as early as the first month of life. Soles and palms may demonstrate well-delineated, painful, progressive hyperkeratotic plaques and papules also associated with hyperhidrosis. There may be severe pain in the soles [69]. Mental retardation occurs in less than 50% of patients. Investigations reveal high urinary and plasma levels of tyrosine, which can be estimated by tandem mass spectrometric assays [66]. It is rarely necessary to perform a liver biopsy to confirm diagnosis.

Ocular Findings

The subjective ocular findings in tyrosinemia type II include conjunctival injection, lacrimation and photophobia. These symptoms can develop as early as at 2 weeks of age [70]. Slit lamp exam reveals deposition of tyrosine crystals in the cornea, resulting in corneal clouding with central or paracentral corneal opacities. Small granular white deposits, arranged in a pseudodendritic pattern in the superficial central cornea of both eyes, may be seen [71]. These patterns have poor staining with fluorescein and rose bengal, and are usually the initial manifestation in patients with tyrosinemia type II [72]. Patients are often misdiagnosed as having recurrent herpes simplex keratitis on presentation until dermatologic manifestations are noticed and tyrosine levels tested [73].

Tyrosinemia Type II versus Schnyder Corneal Dystrophy

While both tyrosinemia type II and SCD are inherited, the former is inherited as an autosomal recessive trait while SCD is autosomal dominant. Both diseases can present at a young age. Patients with tyrosinemia type II have abnormal blood and urinary tyrosine levels while SCD patients do not but frequently have hyperlipidemia. Systemically, the dermatologic and neurologic findings seen in tyrosinemia type II are also not found in SCD. Crystalline deposition in both diseases is superficial but epithelial breakdown, forming pseudodendrites, and scarring only occurs in tyrosinemia type II and is absent in SCD.

Treatment

Studies set a goal to reduce tyrosine blood levels to a maximum of 600 μmol/l. A diet low in tyrosine and alanine has led to a rapid improvement of both ophthalmologic and dermatologic abnormalities [74, 75].

Bietti Crystalline Dystrophy

Definition

Bietti crystalline dystrophy (BCD) is a hereditary disease characterized by the deposition of multiple glistening crystals in the cornea and retina. It is associated with retinal degeneration and sclerosis of the choroidal vessels, which results in progressive night blindness and constriction of the visual fields.

Genetics

BCD is inherited in an autosomal recessive mode and is caused by mutations in the *CYP4V2* gene [76] on chromosome 4q35 [77]. The CYP4V2 protein coded by the *CYP4V2* gene has a similar sequence to other proteins coded by enzymes related to the CYP450 family.

Pathophysiology

Although the pathophysiology of BCD is uncertain, a defect in the CYP4V2 protein is thought to result in abnormal lipid metabolism [78]. This theory is supported by the following findings. Members of the *CYP450* gene family, to which CYP4V2 is related, play a role in the synthesis and digestion of molecules including steroid hormones, bile acids, and certain cholesterols and fatty acids. Additionally, CYP450 enzymes metabolize external substances, such as medications that are ingested, and internal substances, such as toxins that are formed within cells [79]. Corneal and retinal biopsy specimens from more severely affected patients demonstrate crystals resembling cholesterol or cholesterol ester and complex lipid inclusions in corneal, conjunctival, and panchorioretinal fibroblasts [80, 81].

Prevalence

Although patients with BCD have been reported from most parts of the world, the disorder appears to be most common in East Asia, especially in Chinese and Japanese populations. The BCD gene has been estimated to occur at a frequency of 0.005 in China with an average age of onset at 29.3 years [82].

Systemic Findings

Currently there are no abnormal systemic findings reported in BCD.

Ocular Findings

Ophthalmologic lesions normally occur between 20 and 30 years of age [83]. Yellow white punctiform crystals may be found in the superficial and peripheral corneal stroma. These may fade over time. Fundus findings include macular pigment mottling and depigmentation. There may be numerous tiny subretinal refractile yellow dots scattered throughout the posterior pole and the midperiphery associated with diffuse retinal pigment epithelial atrophy and pigment accumulation [83]. With progression, further accumulation of these crystals leads to retinal pigment epithelium atrophy and choroidal sclerosis, seen as confluent loss of choriocapillaris on fluorescein angiogram [84]. These retinal findings are associated with complaints of decreased vision, nyctalopia and peripheral visual field loss [85]. Optical coherence tomography measurements have shown direct correlation between thinning of the retina due to sclerosis and worsening visual acuity [86]. There is progressive loss of the acuity and constriction of the visual fields leading to legal blindness in the fifth to sixth decade [87].

Bietti Crystalline Dystrophy versus Schnyder Corneal Dystrophy

BCD is inherited as an autosomal recessive trait while SCD is inherited as an autosomal dominant trait. BCD demonstrates no systemic lipid abnormalities, while two thirds of SCD patients exhibit hypercholesterolemia. Seventy-five percent of patients with BCD have superficial punctiform corneal crystals while approximately 50% of patients with SCD have superficial crowded needle-like corneal crystals. The crystals in BCD are located at the corneal limbus while those in SCD are located in the central and paracentral cornea. Patients with BCD do not develop arcus lipoides or progressive corneal haze, which are prominent findings in SCD. Nearly all patients with BCD characteristically develop retinal involvement with decreased vision [86], which is not found in SCD.

Treatment

There is currently no treatment for BCD.

Hyperuricemia/Gout

Definition

Hyperuricemia is a heterogeneous group of disorders of purine metabolism that results in increased systemic uric acid. Gout is an abnormality of uric acid metabolism in which there is increased systemic uric acid with deposition of sodium urate crystals in joints, kidneys and soft tissue.

Genetics

There are numerous genetic and environmental factors that can alter systemic uric acid concentrations. Therefore, currently gout has been described to have both a polygenic and monogenic component to its mode of inheritance. Although gout has been shown to run in families, the exact frequency of this is unknown. When familial, gout has an autosomal dominant inheritance that has been mapped to a gene on chromosome 4q25 [88]. In all other cases, there are multiple genes that control the elevated levels of uric acid and thus the inheritance of gout is also variable. One exception is the HGPRT deficiency syndrome which causes hyperuricemia and has an X-linked inheritance pattern [89].

Pathophysiology

A study by Martinon et al. [90] in 2006 demonstrated that in primary gout, monosodium urate and calcium pyrophosphate dihydrate crystals activate the protein inflammasome, which in turn activates interleukin-1β leading to acute inflammation. It was shown that mice lacking components of this pathway exhibited defective inflammatory response. Secondary gout can result from increased uric acid production associated with an acquired metabolic derangement such as myeloproliferative disorders, high purine intake, alcohol consumption, cytotoxic chemotherapy and hypertriglyceridemia. Not all cases of hyperuricemia are associated with the clinical syndrome of gout [91].

Prevalence

The prevalence of gout is 13.6 cases per 1,000 men and 6.4 cases per 1,000 women. Over 90% of gout is found among adult men and 3–7% among postmenopausal women [92].

Systemic Findings

The presentation of gout may be divided into 3 phases, which include asymptomatic hyperuricemia, acute gouty arthritis, and chronic gouty arthritis. About 50% of initial gouty attacks involve the great toe. This type of attack is called podagra, and 90% of patients eventually experience podagra during the course of a lifetime. Another 10% may initially present with polyarticular arthritis [93]. Attacks may be precipitated by various stresses such as dietary, physical and emotional. Chronic gouty arthritis causes progressive inability to dispose of urate, which causes further deposition in cartilage, tendons, and soft tissue forming tophi [94]. Tophaceous deposits produce irregular swelling and lead to destruction of joint spaces. Patients with gout are also more likely, by a factor of 1,000, to develop renal stones and may have a history of renal colic [95]. Indeed, renal stones may precede the onset of gout in 40% of affected patients. While 80% of these patients may have stones composed entirely of uric acid, 20% may develop calcium oxalate or calcium phosphate stones with a uric acid core [95].

Ocular Findings

Urate crystals may deposit in the conjunctiva [96], sclera, cornea, iris, anterior chamber, lens, tarsal cartilage and tendons of extraocular muscles [97]. One study showed the most common ocular finding to be hyperemia and dilated tortuous conjunctival vessels, which was reported in 62% of patients [98]. Conjunctivitis and episcleritis has also been noted [99]. Only 2% of patients demonstrated attacks of scleritis. Although rare, isolated corneal deposits of uric acid crystals are found in the superficial stroma and epithelium [96]. They can span the intrapalpebral limbal area adjacent to episcleral vessels [99]. With the presence of band keratopathy, the yellow-tinted crystals have also been described in the deep corneal epithelial cells and at the level of the Bowman membrane [96]. Band keratopathy seen with gouty arthritis cannot be distinguished from typical calcific band keratopathy. Histopathologic examination reveals that the needle-like crystals are located within the nuclei of corneal epithelial cells and have negative birefringence [100].

Gout versus Schnyder Corneal Dystrophy

While the major systemic finding in gout is hyperuricemia, the major systemic finding in two thirds of patients with SCD is hypercholesterolemia. Although unclear, gout does not usually have a familial history, while SCD is almost always inherited in an autosomal dominant fashion. The crystals in gout show deposition in many ocular tissues including the sclera and conjunctiva while SCD crystalline deposits are confined to the cornea. These crystals are found in rare instances in gout while they are commonly found in SCD where they present in approximately half of the patients with SCD. The location of the crystals in SCD is anterior subepithelial, which is similar to gout; however, their central location differs from gouty crystals which are deposited near the limbus adjacent to episcleral vessels. The histopathology of the crystals also differs. Those in gout demonstrate uric acid whereas those in SCD demonstrate lipid.

Treatment

For urate crystals within the ocular tissue, treatment is directed at reducing both hyperuricemia and ocular inflammation. Moderate reduction of purine in diet can help reduce both the frequency and the severity of attacks of gout. Medical treatment involves hydration, colchicine for prevention and acute treatment, nonsteroidal and steroidal anti-inflammatory drugs. Uricosuric and antihyperuricemic drugs, such as probenecid and allopurinol, respectively, are effective in treatment [101].

Multiple Myeloma/Monoclonal Gammopathy

Definition

Multiple myeloma and benign monoclonal gammopathy of unknown significance (MGUS) are characterized by an abnormal proliferation of malignant plasma cells with resultant excess accumulation of monoclonal paraprotein. While myeloma is considered a malignant disease, MGUS is considered a benign or possibly a premyelomatous condition [102].

Genetics

Although the exact cause remains unknown, MGUS and multiple myeloma are thought to arise due to an abnormal translocations involving the immunoglobulin heavy-chain gene at 14q32 along with deletions of the long arm of chromosome 13 [103, 104].

Pathophysiology

Multiple myeloma is caused by a monoclonal proliferation of plasma cells with overproduction of antibody light (kappa or lamda) and heavy chains, leading to hyperviscosity, amyloidosis, and renal failure. Accompanying findings include leukopenia, anemia, thrombocytopenia, soft-tissue masses called plasmacytomas and skeletal lytic lesions. The aberrant antibodies produced lead to impaired humoral immunity resulting in increased frequency of infection, especially with encapsulated organisms such as *Pneumococcus*.

Prevalence

Approximately 1 in 4,317 or 0.02% or 63,000 people in the United States are affected by multiple myeloma. An estimated 19,920 new cases of multiple myeloma were diagnosed in 2008. Of these, about 11,190 were men and 8,730 were women. Multiple myeloma is slightly more common among men than women, and almost twice as common among blacks as among whites. The average age at diagnosis is 65–70 years.

Systemic Findings

Systemic findings in multiple myeloma include pathologic fractures, anemia, infection, hypercalcemia, spinal cord compression, or renal failure. Hypercalcemia is found in 30% of patients [105] and may present with confusion, somnolence, constipation, nausea, and thirst. Bone pain of the lumbar spine, which may proceed to pathologic fractures, is the most common symptom in multiple myeloma presenting in 70% of patients at diagnosis. This can lead to spinal cord compression in approximately 10–20% of cases [106]. The most common cause of weakness at disease presentation is anemia. Blood hyperviscosity in high tumor volume can also increase chances and complications of stroke, myocardial ischemia, or infarction [107].

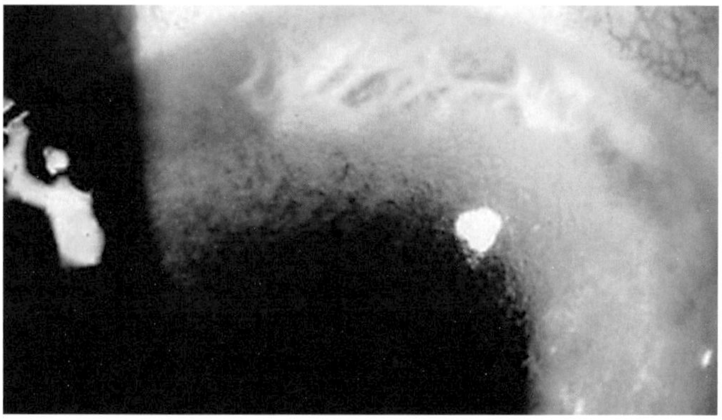

Fig. 5. Diffuse peripheral corneal deposits seen in a patient with multiple myeloma. Source: http://www.atlasophthalmology.com/atlas/photo.jsf?node=4218&locale=en (online atlas of ophthalmology).

Unlike multiple myeloma, MGUS does not cause systemic symptoms in most people and is found by accident on blood tests when patients are checked for other conditions.

Ocular Findings

Crystalline keratopathy occurs only rarely in association with multiple myeloma and monoclonal gammopathy [108]. In both cases, the crystals are commonly composed of IgG light chains [109] and may be found to be deposited both within and in between cells of corneal epithelium and anterior stroma [110–112].

Diffuse superficial punctiform crystals may be found in the central and peripheral cornea [113] (fig. 5). Additional fleck-like corneal haze may be present. Patients with corneal immunoglobulin deposition most frequently complain of photophobia; however, visual acuity is typically spared [113]. Cysts of the ciliary body and retinal vascular lesions have also been reported in multiple myeloma patients [114].

In monoclonal gammopathy, corneal deposits studied with an electron microscopy show that the electron-dense deposits are composed of parallel fine filaments [115, 116]. They are tubular crystalloid deposits with a central lucent core [117]. The deposition of these crystals may cause damage and decrease the number of keratocytes and corneal endothelial cells [118].

Of note, studies have shown that hypercupremia may occur with bilateral copper deposits in the Descemet membrane, iris surface, and lens capsule in both multiple myeloma and MGUS [119, 120].

Multiple Myeloma/Monoclonal Gammopathy of Unknown Significance versus Schnyder Corneal Dystrophy

The prominent systemic finding in multiple myeloma/MGUS is immunoglobulin overproduction, leading to hematologic and other systemic abnormalities, whereas the main systemic presentation of SCD is hyperlipidemia. In those SCD patients with crowded needle-like crystals, these are confined to the central and paracentral cornea and may be large or small with an irregular pattern. By contrast, the crystals in multiple myeloma/MGUS are small, punctiform and can extend to the limbus. While both multiple myeloma/MGUS patients and SCD patients may complain of photophobia with crystalline deposits, by middle age, photophobia and loss of photopic vision often become visually disabling in SCD unlike in multiple myeloma/MGUS. Finally, potential additional ocular findings of ciliary body cysts and corneal copper deposits in multiple myeloma/MGUS are not found in SCD.

Treatment
A large study demonstrated that 19% of 241 patients with a diagnosis of benign monoclonal gammopathy developed myeloma, or a related disorder, when followed for 10 years or more [121]. The mortality rate of multiple myeloma remains high. Reports have shown that myeloma-associated crystalline keratopathy can disappear in response to chemotherapy and plasma exchange [111, 112].

Infectious Crystalline Keratopathy

Definition
Infectious crystalline keratopathy (ICK) is characterized by white, branching, crystalline opacities within the corneal stroma with little or no associated inflammatory response [122].

Pathophysiology
ICK is caused by indolent and fastidious organisms which become implanted in the corneal stroma in a setting of immunosuppression such as from corticosteroid use, contact lens wear, or infected corneal grafts. Histopathologic examination of corneal buttons has demonstrated pockets of bacteria between corneal lamellae and little inflammatory reaction [123].

Etiology/Prevalence
Studies have shown the most cultured organisms in ICK to be the *Streptococcus* species, with α-hemolytic *Streptococcus* being the most common [122, 124]. ICK may also be associated with culture-proven *Streptococcus pneumoniae* [125], *Haemophilus species* [126], *Pseudomonas aeruginosa* [127], *Gemella haemolysans* [123], *Candida* and *Alternaria* fungi [128], as well as *Acanthamoeba* [129].

One large study spanning from 1978 to 1995 reported on 18 eyes with ICK and found 55% to be caused by Gram-positive cocci, 28% by Gram-negative rods, and 17% by fungi [124].

Ocular Findings
The most common presentation of ICK occurs in an uninflamed corneal graft as a slowly growing, sharply demarcated, snowflake-like stromal opacity [130]. Although

commonly stromal, the crystalline opacities may be present in any layer of the cornea [131]. Electron microscopy reveals a characteristic trilamellar structure of bacterial cell walls and small electron-dense bodies with needle-like projections [132]. Although uncertain, these bodies may be responsible for the crystalline appearance of this keratopathy.

Infectious Crystalline Keratopathy versus Schnyder Corneal Dystrophy
Although ICK is responsible for causing crystalline deposits in the corneal stroma, there are numerous differences that separate it from SCD. ICK is an infection seen most commonly after corneal transplants and is an acquired condition whereas SCD is an autosomal dominant inherited disease. The location of crystal deposition in ICK can be seen throughout the corneal stroma and epithelium; however, those of SCD are only within the subepithelial space. Clinically, ICK exhibits the classic snowflake-like opacity against a clear background and lacks any arcus lipoides and midstromal haze seen with SCD.

Treatment
Treatment initially consists of cessation of topical steroids and prolonged use of topical bactericidal antibiotics. It is recommended starting with vancomycin or another potent antibiotic with good Gram-positive coverage and adapting medications depending on culture or biopsy results. Some authors suggest systemic antibiotics in severe and fungal cases [133]. Regardless, ICK is extremely difficult to treat, demonstrating poor and slow response to medications. Debilitating stromal scars or recurrence of infections are common. In many cases, despite appropriate antimicrobial therapy, repeat penetrating keratoplasty or lamellar keratectomy may be required [134, 135].

Dieffenbachia Keratitis

Definition
Dieffenbachia keratitis occurs due to an ocular injury from exposure to the *Dieffenbachia* plant which is a tropical house plant belonging to the Araceae family [136].

Pathophysiology
Keratitis is instigated after the stem or branches of the plant are broken. This is followed by an explosive release of fluid containing needle-like crystals of calcium oxalate (raphides). If struck with the plant or fluid, the calcium oxalate crystals may penetrate the cornea [137].

Systemic Findings
None.

Ocular Findings
After ocular injury with the *Dieffenbachia* plant, patients may complain of pain, burning and conjunctival injection. Visual acuity is usually not affected [137]. Conjunctival swelling and iritis may follow. The corneal crystals appear as numerous and highly reflective. They have an elongated needle-shaped structure [138]. Slit lamp biomicroscopy demonstrates fine punctate opacities of calcium oxalate crystals that can be seen to span all layers of the corneal stroma diffusely.

Dieffenbachia Keratitis versus Schnyder Corneal Dystrophy
Dieffenbachia keratitis is associated with ocular injury while SCD usually has a history of autosomal dominant inheritance. Systemic hypercholesterolemia is found in over 2/3 of SCD patients but is not found in Dieffenbachia keratitis [6]. The raphides crystals may be found in any layer of the cornea unlike SCD crystals, which are only found in the subepithelium. There is no corneal haze or arcus lipoides in Dieffenbachia keratitis. In SCD, arcus lipoides and progressive corneal haze are prominent findings in the disease. All patients aged 23 years and older have arcus lipoides. Injury with *Dieffenbachia* plant resolves with time while corneal changes with SCD are progressive.

Treatment
Patients may be treated with light topical steroids [137] and corneal crystals have been shown to vanish within about 3 weeks after presentation [139].

Gold

Pathophysiology
Systemic gold therapy is used for the treatment of collagen vascular diseases, such as Sjögren's syndrome, lupus erythematosus, and particularly rheumatoid arthritis. The deposition of gold in the cornea is termed corneal chrysiasis. This occurs when the cumulative dose of the medication taken exceeds 1,500 mg [140]. During the course of treatment, the concentration of gold in the cornea is found to be elevated when compared to other tissues and the duration of chrysotherapy correlates directly with the clinical density of deposits [141].

Ocular Findings
Gold may deposit in the aqueous humor, iris, ciliary body, and in all layers of the cornea [142, 143]. The natural flow of gold particles within the aqueous humor results in inferior corneal depositions while the superior and peripheral cornea are spared [141]. The gold particles appear as yellow-brown dots which may have a metallic sheen. Although the deposits have the potential of clearing after therapy is stopped, some deposits may persist for years [144].

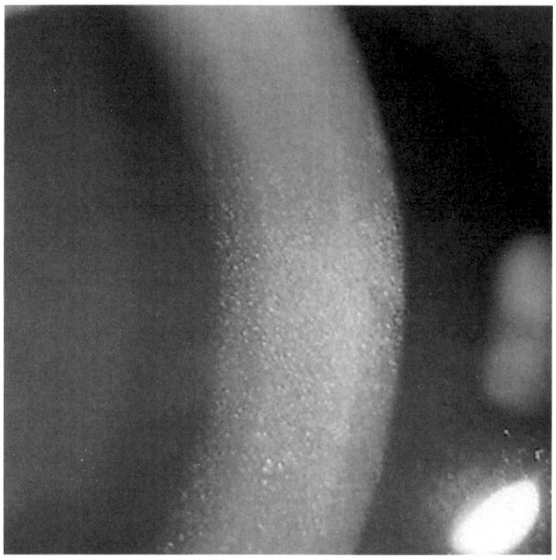

Fig. 6. Small creamy-white deposits seen concentrated in posterior corneal layers with chlorpromazine deposition. Source: http://www.atlasophthalmology.com/atlas/photo.jsf?node=4642& locale=en (online atlas of ophthalmology).

Chrysiasis versus Schnyder Corneal Dystrophy

Although chrysiasis and SCD both have abnormal corneal deposits, there are numerous differences that distinguish the 2 entities. In the patient with chrysiasis, history will reveal medical treatment with gold for autoimmune disease. In SCD, there is autosomal dominant inheritance with a frequent history of hyperlipidemia. Slit lamp examination in chrysiasis may reveal gold deposits in the posterior stroma and Descemet membrane while crystalline deposition in SCD is in the corneal subepithelium. Only SCD patients demonstrate the progressive corneal haze and arcus lipoides.

Chlorpromazine

Pathophysiology

Chlorpromazine is the oldest prescribed antipsychotic, often used in the treatment of bipolar disorder or schizophrenia. Patients who take chlorpromazine for extended periods of time, with doses exceeding 400 mg/day or 1,100 g in total, have been shown to develop bilateral corneal crystalline deposition [145, 146].

Ocular Findings

Slit lamp biomicroscopy reveals multiple fine creamy-white deposits in the cornea and anterior crystalline lens capsule bilaterally (fig. 6). In vivo confocal microscopy has identified irregular hyperreflective deposits on the posterior surface of the corneal endothelium. The deposits range from 1 to 70 μm in diameter, have well-defined edges [146], and may cause corneal endothelial cell pleomorphism and polymegethism [147]. There may be reduction in visual acuity, but it is typically minimal ranging from 20/30 to 20/60 [146]. Light exposure may result in cellular damage particularly because chlorpromazine is a phototoxic compound. Consequently, once corneal crystals are noted to occur, chlorpromazine treatment should be stopped.

Chlorpromazine versus Schnyder Corneal Dystrophy
History should reveal the presence of a psychiatric disease treated with chlorpromazine. In SCD, a family history typically reveals autosomal dominance. Hyperlipidemia is frequent in SCD but not associated with the use of chlorpromazine. One of the main differences between the 2 entities is the location of the deposits. In chlorpromazine therapy, they are found in the posterior cornea affecting endothelial cells, whereas crystalline deposits in SCD are anterior, subepithelial, and associated with progressive corneal haze.

Chloroquine

Pathophysiology
Chloroquine is used in the treatment or prevention of malaria and as a mild immunosuppressor in the treatment of autoimmune disorders such as rheumatoid arthritis and lupus erythematosus. Chloroquine is a lysomotropic agent, which causes its accumulation preferentially in the lysosomes of cells in the body [148].

Ocular Findings
The ocular manifestations of chloroquine-associated ocular disease include a reversible anterior keratopathy and an irreversible retinopathy. The bilateral keratopathy appears months after drug use and has been reported at cumulative levels as low as 400 g. One study showed that 50% of patients exhibited deposits when nearing a total dose of 1,250 g [149]. These deposits can be eliminated after cessation of the drug [150]. Although corneal changes do not cause a decrease in visual acuity, complaints of halos have been reported. In vivo confocal microscopy demonstrated that the deposits are highly reflective, dot-like intracellular inclusions concentrated in the basal epithelial layers and anterior stroma [151]. These cells have a concentrically lamellated configuration and appear consistent with intralysosomal lipid accumulation seen with chloroquine therapy. In contrast with retinopathy, the presence of the keratopathy is not an indication to stop treatment [152].

Chloroquine versus Schnyder Corneal Dystrophy
History should reveal risk or treatment of malaria or autoimmune disease if a patient has chloroquine corneal crystals. In SCD, autosomal dominant inheritance is typical in addition to hyperlipidemia, which occurs in the majority of patients. Both chloroquine keratopathy and SCD can have crystalline deposition in the anterior corneal stroma. The usual arcus lipoides and midperipheral haze present in SCD are lacking

in chloroquine keratopathy. Also, cessation of chloroquine medication can reverse corneal deposits whereas those in SCD are progressive.

Clofazimine

Pathophysiology

Clofazimine is a fat-soluble riminophenazine used in combination with rifampin and dapsone as multidrug therapy for the treatment of leprosy. Clofazimine has a very long half-life of about 70 days and autopsies have found crystallized clofazimine in the intestinal mucosa, liver, spleen, and corneal tissue [153].

Ocular Findings

Ocular involvement includes depositions of reddish brown conjunctival and corneal pigmentation, which have been seen in as many as 46 and 53% of the patients, respectively [154]. One study showed these changes to be present after 3 years of therapy at a dose of 100 mg twice daily. Slit lamp examination can show myriad polychromatic crystals diffusely involving the cornea in all layers and perilimbal conjunctiva of both eyes. A biopsy of conjunctival tissue showed numerous rectangular- or rhomboidal-shaped crystals within stromal fibroblasts and macrophages. Additionally, complex lipid inclusions were observed in mesenchymal cells as well as in endothelial cells and pericytes of blood vessels [155]. Fortunately, in most cases, there are no functional changes in visual acuity and changes are reversible after cessation of medication [156].

Clofazimine versus Schnyder Corneal Dystrophy

There are many differences which separate clofazimine keratopathy from SCD. Patients with clofazimine keratopathy usually have a history of leprosy, whereas SCD patients have a familial history with autosomal dominance. The reddish brown pigmentation described with clofazimine therapy can be clearly distinguished from the whitish crystalline deposits that may occur in SCD. Clofazimine may deposit in any layer of the cornea, while SCD crystals typically occur in the subepithelium. Also, clofazimine therapy lacks progressive corneal haze and arcus lipoides seen in SCD and may be reversible with discontinuation of the drug.

References

1 Theendakara V, Tromp G, Kuivaniemi H, et al: Fine mapping of the schnyder's crystalline corneal dystrophy locus. Hum Genet 2004;114:594–600.

2 Weiss JS, Kruth HS, Kuivaniemi H, et al: Mutations in the UBIAD1 gene on chromosome short arm 1, region 36, cause schnyder crystalline corneal dystrophy. Invest Ophthalmol Vis Sci 2007;48:5007–5012.

3 Orr A, Dube MP, Marcadier J, Jiang H, Federico A, George S, Seamone C, Andrews D, Dubord P, Holland S: Mutations in the UBIAD1 gene, encoding a potential prenyltransferase, are causal for schnyder crystalline corneal dystrophy. PLoS One 2007;2:e685.
4 Shearman AM, Hudson TJ, Andresen JM, et al: The gene for schnyder's crystalline corneal dystrophy maps to human chromosome 1p34.1-p36. Hum Mol Genet 1996;5:1667–1672.
5 Gaynor PM, Zhang WY, Weiss JS, et al: Accumulation of HDL apolipoproteins accompanies abnormal cholesterol accumulation in schnyder's corneal dystrophy. Arterioscler Thromb Vasc Biol 1996;16: 992–999.
6 Weiss JS: Visual morbidity in thirty-four families with schnyder crystalline corneal dystrophy (an American Ophthalmological Society thesis). Trans Am Ophthalmol Soc 2007;105:616–648.
7 Brownstein S, Jackson WB, Onerheim RM: Schnyder's crystalline corneal dystrophy in association with hyperlipoproteinemia: histopathological and ultrastructural findings. Can J Ophthalmol 1991;26:273–279.
8 Bron AJ: Corneal changes in the dislipoproteinaemias. Cornea 1989;8:135–140.
9 McCarthy M, Innis S, Dubord P, White V: Panstromal schnyder corneal dystrophy. A clinical pathologic report with quantitative analysis of corneal lipid composition. Ophthalmology 1994; 101:895–901.
10 Lisch W, Weidle EG, Lisch C, et al: Schnyder's dystrophy. Progression and metabolism. Ophthalmic Paediatr Genet 1986;7:45–56.
11 Barchiesi BJ, Eckel RH, Ellis PP: The cornea and disorders of lipid metabolism. Surv Ophthalmol 1991;36:1–22.
12 Bron AJ, Williams HP, Carruthers ME: Hereditary crystalline stromal dystrophy of Schnyder. I. Clinical features of a family with hyperlipoproteinaemia. Br J Ophthalmol 1972;56:383–399.
13 Hoang-Xuan T, Pouliquen Y, Savoldelli M, Gasteau J: Schnyder's crystalline dystrophy. I. Study of a case by light and electron microscopy. J Fr Ophtalmol 1985;8:735–742.
14 Hoang-Xuan T, Pouliquen Y, Gasteau J: Schnyder's crystalline dystrophy. II. Association with genu valgum. J Fr Ophtalmol 1985;8:743–747.
15 Weiss JS: Schnyder's dystrophy of the cornea. A swede-finn connection. Cornea 1992;11:93–101.
16 Ciancaglini M, Carpineto P, Doronzo E, et al: Morphological evaluation of schnyder's central crystalline dystrophy by confocal microscopy before and after phototherapeutic keratectomy. J Cataract Refract Surg 2001;27:1892–1895.
17 Jing Y, Wang L: Morphological evaluation of schnyder's crystalline corneal dystrophy by laser scanning confocal microscopy and fourier-domain optical coherence tomography. Clin Experiment Ophthalmol 2009;37:308–312.
18 Weiss JS, Rodrigues MM, Kruth HS, et al: Panstromal schnyder's corneal dystrophy. Ultrastructural and histochemical studies. Ophthalmology 1992;99:1072–1081.
19 Jonas A: Lecithin cholesterol acyltransferase. Biochim Biophys Acta 2000;1529:245–256.
20 Norum KR, Gjone E: Familial serum-cholesterol esterification failure. A new inborn error of metabolism. Biochim Biophys Acta 1967;144:698–700.
21 Horl G, Kroisel PM, Wagner E, et al: Compound heterozygosity (G71R/R140H) in the lecithin: cholesterol acyltransferase (LCAT) gene results in an intermediate phenotype between LCAT-deficiency and fish-eye disease. Atherosclerosis 2006;187:101–109.
22 McLean J, Fielding C, Drayna D, et al: Cloning and expression of human lecithin-cholesterol acyltransferase cDNA. Proc Natl Acad Sci USA 1986; 83:2335–2339.
23 Azoulay M, Henry I, Tata F, et al: The structural gene for lecithin:cholesterol acyl transferase (LCAT) maps to 16q22. Ann Hum Genet 1987;51: 129–136.
24 Kralovicova J, Lei H, Vorechovsky I: Phenotypic consequences of branch point substitutions. Hum Mutat 2006;27:803–813.
25 Alawadhi M, Thanassoulis G, Marcil M, Genest J: Genetic lipoprotein disorders and coronary atherosclerosis. Curr Atheroscler Rep 2005;7:196–203.
26 Funke H, von Eckardstein A, Pritchard PH, et al: Genetic and phenotypic heterogeneity in familial lecithin: cholesterol acyltransferase (LCAT) deficiency. Six newly identified defective alleles further contribute to the structural heterogeneity in this disease. J Clin Invest 1993;91:677–683.
27 Weidle EG, Lisch W: Corneal opacity as the leading symptom of hereditary lecithin-cholesterol acyltransferase (LCAT) deficiency. Case report and a review of the literature. Klin Monatsbl Augenheilkd 1987;190:182–187.
28 Schmidt HH, Diekstall FF, Bojanovski D, Manns MP: Fish eye disease. Dtsch Med Wochenschr 1994; 119:1393–1396.
29 Clerc M, Pouliquen Y: Arcus juvenilis and lecithin:cholesterol acyltransferase functions. Report of a case of familial fish-eye-disease. Bull Acad Natl Med 1993;177:807–820.
30 McIntyre N: Familial LCAT deficiency and fish-eye disease. J Inherit Metab Dis 1988;11(suppl 1): 45–56.

31 Chu FC, Kuwabara T, Cogan DG, Schaefer EJ, Brewer HB: Ocular manifestations of familial high-density lipoprotein deficiency (Tangier disease). Arch Ophthalmol 1979;97:1926–1928.
32 Frohlich J, Hoag G, McLeod R, et al: Hypoalphalipoproteinemia resembling fish eye disease. Acta Med Scand 1987;221:291–298.
33 Kastelein JJ, Pritchard PH, Erkelens DW, et al: Familial high-density-lipoprotein deficiency causing corneal opacities (fish eye disease) in a family of dutch descent. J Intern Med 1992;231:413–419.
34 Carlson LA: Fish eye disease: a new familial condition with massive corneal opacities and dyslipoproteinaemia. Eur J Clin Invest 1982;12:41–43.
35 Clerc M, Dumon MF, Sess D, et al: A 'Fish-eye disease' familial condition with massive corneal opacities and hypoalphalipoproteinaemia: clinical, biochemical and genetic features. Eur J Clin Invest 1991;21:616–624.
36 Kohnen T, Pelton RW, Jones DB: Schnyder corneal dystrophy and juvenile, systemic hypercholesteremia. Klin Monatsbl Augenheilkd 1997;211:135–137.
37 Borven I, Egge K, Gjone E: Corneal and fundus changes in familial LCAT-deficiency. Acta Ophthalmol (Copenh) 1974;52:201–210.
38 Berard AM, Clerc M, Brewer B, Santamarina-Fojo S: A normal rate of cellular cholesterol removal can be mediated by plasma from a patient with familial lecithin-cholesterol acyltransferase (LCAT) deficiency. Clin Chim Acta 2001;314:131–139.
39 De Smedt M, Van Ginderdeuren R, De Vos R, et al: Corneal opacifications in a low high density lipoprotein syndrome: suspicion of fish eye disease: a case report. Bull Soc Belge Ophtalmol 2001:25–30.
40 Herrmann WA, von Mohrenfels CW, Lohmann CP: Confocal microscopy and corneal sensitivity in a patient with corneal manifestations of Tangier disease. Cornea 2004;23:825–827.
41 Rust S, Rosier M, Funke H, et al: Tangier disease is caused by mutations in the gene encoding ATP-binding cassette transporter 1. Nat Genet 1999;22: 352–355.
42 Rust S, Walter M, Funke H, et al: Assignment of tangier disease to chromosome 9q31 by a graphical linkage exclusion strategy. Nat Genet 1998;20: 96–98.
43 Remaley AT, Rust S, Rosier M, et al: Human ATP-binding cassette transporter 1 (ABC1): genomic organization and identification of the genetic defect in the original tangier disease kindred. Proc Natl Acad Sci U S A 1999;96:12685–12690.
44 Pietrini V, Rizzuto N, Vergani C, et al: Neuropathy in tangier disease: A clinicopathologic study and a review of the literature. Acta Neurol Scand 1985; 72:495–505.
45 Schippling S, Orth M, Beisiegel U, et al: Severe tangier disease with a novel ABCA1 gene mutation. Neurology 2008;71:1454–1454.
46 Brooks-Wilson A, Marcil M, Clee SM, et al: Mutations in ABC1 in tangier disease and familial high-density lipoprotein deficiency. Nat Genet 1999;22:336-345.
47 Schaefer EJ, Zech LA, Schwartz DE, Brewer HB: Coronary heart disease prevalence and other clinical features in familial high-density lipoprotein deficiency (Tangier disease). Ann Intern Med 1980; 93:261–266.
48 Pressly TA, Scott WJ, Ide CH, et al: Ocular complications of tangier disease. Am J Med 1987;83: 991–994.
49 Chu FC, Kuwabara T, Cogan DG, et al: Ocular manifestations of familial high-density lipoprotein deficiency (tangier disease). Arch Ophthalmol 1979;97: 1926–1928.
50 Schneider JA, Bradley K, Seegmiller JE: Increased cystine in leukocytes from individuals homozygous and heterozygous for cystinosis. Science 1967;157: 1321–1322.
51 Kalatzis V, Cherqui S, Antignac C, Gasnier B: Cystinosin, the protein defective in cystinosis, is a H(+)-driven lysosomal cystine transporter. EMBO J 2001;20:5940–5949.
52 Attard M, Jean G, Forestier L, et al: Severity of phenotype in cystinosis varies with mutations in the CTNS gene: predicted effect on the model of cystinosin. Hum Mol Genet 1999;8:2507–2514.
53 Kalatzis V, Nevo N, Cherqui S, et al: Molecular pathogenesis of cystinosis: effect of CTNS mutations on the transport activity and subcellular localization of cystinosin. Hum Mol Genet 2004;13: 1361–1371.
54 Kleta R, Anikster Y, Lucero C, et al: CTNS mutations in african american patients with cystinosis. Mol Genet Metab 2001;74:332–337.
55 Bois E, Feingold J, Frenay P, Briard ML: Infantile cystinosis in france: genetics, incidence, geographic distribution. J Med Genet 1976;13:434–438.
56 Wen SF, Friedman AL, Oberley TD: Two case studies from a family with primary Fanconi syndrome. Am J Kidney Dis 1989;13:240–246.
57 Gahl WA, Thoene JG, Schneider JA: Cystinosis. N Engl J Med 2002;347:111–121.
58 Katz B, Melles RB, Schneider JA: Contrast sensitivity function in nephropathic cystinosis. Arch Ophthalmol 1987;105:1667–1669.
59 Labbe A, Niaudet P, Loirat C, et al: In vivo confocal microscopy and anterior segment optical coherence tomography analysis of the cornea in nephropathic cystinosis. Ophthalmology 2009;116:870–876.

60 Gahl WA, Kuehl EM, Iwata F, et al: Corneal crystals in nephropathic cystinosis: natural history and treatment with cysteamine eyedrops. Mol Genet Metab 2000;71:100–120.

61 Brubaker RF, Wong VG, Schulman JD, et al: Benign cystinosis. The clinical, biochemical and morphologic findings in a family with two affected siblings. Am J Med 1970;49:546–550.

62 Tsilou ET, Rubin BI, Reed G, et al: Nephropathic cystinosis: posterior segment manifestations and effects of cysteamine therapy. Ophthalmology 2006; 113:1002–1009.

63 Kimonis VE, Troendle J, Rose SR, et al: Effects of early cysteamine therapy on thyroid function and growth in nephropathic cystinosis. J Clin Endocrinol Metab 1995;80:3257–3261.

64 Kaiser-Kupfer MI, Fujikawa L, Kuwabara T, et al: Removal of corneal crystals by topical cysteamine in nephropathic cystinosis. N Engl J Med 1987;316: 775–779.

65 da Silva VA, Zurbrugg RP, Lavanchy P, et al: Long-term treatment of infantile nephropathic cystinosis with cysteamine. N Engl J Med 1985;313: 1460–1463.

66 Tallab TM: Richner-Hanhart syndrome importance of early diagnosis and early intervention. J Am Acad Dermatol 1996;35:857–859.

67 Hanhart E: [Not Available]. Dermatologica 1947;94: 286–308.

68 Fellman JH, Vanbellinghen PJ, Jones RT, Koler RD: Soluble and mitochondrial forms of tyrosine aminotransferase. Relationship to human tyrosinemia. Biochemistry 1969;8:615–622.

69 Rabinowitz LG, Williams LR, Anderson CE, et al: Painful keratoderma and photophobia: hallmarks of tyrosinemia type II. J Pediatr 1995;126:266–269.

70 Goldsmith LA: Tyrosinemia II. Int J Dermatol 1985; 24:293–294.

71 Tsai CP, Lin PY, Lee NC, et al: Corneal lesion as the initial manifestation of tyrosinemia type II. J Chin Med Assoc 2006;69:286–288.

72 Macsai MS, Schwartz TL, Hinkle D, et al: Tyrosinemia type II: nine cases of ocular signs and symptoms. Am J Ophthalmol 2001;132:522–527.

73 al-Hemidan AI, al-Hazzaa SA: Richner-hanhart syndrome (tyrosinemia type II). Case report and literature review. Ophthalmic Genet 1995;16:21–26.

74 Machino H, Miki Y, Kawatsu T, et al: Successful dietary control of tyrosinemia II. J Am Acad Dermatol 1983;9:533–539.

75 Godde-Jolly D, Larregue M, Roussat B, Van Effenterre G: A case of richner-hanhart syndrome (tyrosinosis with ocular, cutaneous and mental manifestations. J Fr Ophtalmol 1979;2:23–28.

76 Li A, Jiao X, Munier FL, et al: Bietti crystalline corneoretinal dystrophy is caused by mutations in the novel gene CYP4V2. Am J Hum Genet 2004;74: 817–826.

77 Jiao X, Munier FL, Iwata F, et al: Genetic linkage of bietti crystallin corneoretinal dystrophy to chromosome 4q35. Am J Hum Genet 2000;67: 1309–1313.

78 Lee J, Jiao X, Hejtmancik JF, et al: The metabolism of fatty acids in human bietti crystalline dystrophy. Invest Ophthalmol Vis Sci 2001;42:1707–1714.

79 Nakano M, Kelly EJ, Rettie AE: Expression and characterization of CYP4V2 as a fatty acid {omega}-hydroxylase. Drug Metab Dispos 2009.

80 Kaiser-Kupfer MI, Chan CC, Markello TC, et al: Clinical biochemical and pathologic correlations in bietti's crystalline dystrophy. Am J Ophthalmol 1994;118:569–582.

81 Harrison RJ, Acheson RR, Dean-Hart JC: Bietti's tapetoretinal degeneration with marginal corneal dystrophy (crystalline retinopathy): Case report. Br J Ophthalmol 1987;71:220–223.

82 Hu D-N: Ophthalmic genetics in china. Ophthal Paediat Genet 1983;2:39–45.

83 Chaker N, Mghaieth F, Baccouri R, et al: Clinical and angiographic characteristics of Bietti's corneoretinal dystrophy: A case study of an 8-year-old girl. J Fr Ophtalmol 2007;30:39–43.

84 Fong AM, Koh A, Lee K, Ang CL: Bietti's crystalline dystrophy in Asians: Clinical, angiographic and electrophysiological characteristics. Int Ophthalmol 2008.

85 Meyer CH, Rodrigues EB, Mennel S, Schmidt JC: Optical coherence tomography in a case of Bietti's crystalline dystrophy. Acta Ophthalmol Scand 2004; 82:609–612.

86 Lai TY, Ng TK, Tam PO, et al: Genotype phenotype analysis of bietti's crystalline dystrophy in patients with CYP4V2 mutations. Invest Ophthalmol Vis Sci 2007;48:5212–5220.

87 Bernauer W, Daicker B: Bietti's corneal-retinal dystrophy. A 16-year progression. Retina 1992;12:18–20.

88 Cheng LS, Chiang SL, Tu HP, et al: Genomewide scan for gout in taiwanese aborigines reveals linkage to chromosome 4q25. Am J Hum Genet 2004;75: 498–503.

89 Hoefnagel D, Andrew ED, Mireault NG, Berndt WO: Hereditary choreoathetosis, self-mutilation and hyperuricemia in young males. N Engl J Med 1965;273:130–135.

90 Martinon F, Petrilli V, Mayor A, et al: Gout-associated uric acid crystals activate the NALP3 inflammasome. Nature 2006;440:237–241.

91 Liote F, Ea HK: Recent developments in crystal-induced inflammation pathogenesis and management. Curr Rheumatol Rep 2007;9:243–250.
92 Meyers OL, Monteagudo FS: Gout in females: an analysis of 92 patients. Clin Exp Rheumatol 1985;3: 105–109.
93 Puig JG, Michan AD, Jimenez ML, et al: Female gout. Clinical spectrum and uric acid metabolism. Arch Intern Med 1991;151:726–732.
94 Akahoshi T, Murakami Y, Kitasato H: Recent advances in crystal-induced acute inflammation. Curr Opin Rheumatol 2007;19:146–150.
95 Wallace SL, Singer JZ, Duncan GJ, et al: Renal function predicts colchicine toxicity: guidelines for the prophylactic use of colchicine in gout. J Rheumatol 1991;18:264–269.
96 Lo WR, Broocker G, Grossniklaus HE: Histopathologic examination of conjunctival tophi in gouty arthritis. Am J Ophthalmol 2005;140: 1152–1154.
97 Coassin M, Piovanetti O, Stark WJ, Green WR: Urate deposition in the iris and anterior chamber. Ophthalmology 2006;113:462–465.
98 Ferry AP, Safir A, Melikian HE: Ocular abnormalities in patients with gout. Ann Ophthalmol 1985;17: 632–635.
99 Bernad B, Narvaez J, Diaz-Torne C, et al: Clinical image: corneal tophus deposition in gout. Arthritis Rheum 2006;54:1025.
100 Slansky HH, Kubara T: Intranuclear urate crystals in corneal epithelium. Arch Ophthalmol 1968;80: 338–844.
101 Terkeltaub R: Gout. Novel therapies for treatment of gout and hyperuricemia. Arthritis Res Ther 2009; 11:236.
102 Orellana J, Friedman AH: Ocular manifestations of multiple myeloma, Waldenstrom's macroglobulinemia and benign monoclonal gammopathy. Surv Ophthalmol 1981;26:157–169.
103 Harrison CJ, Mazzullo H, Ross FM, et al: Translocations of 14q32 and deletions of 13q14 are common chromosomal abnormalities in systemic amyloidosis. Br J Haematol 2002;117: 427–435.
104 Takimoto M, Ogawa K, Kato Y, et al: Close relation between 14q32/IGH translocations and chromosome 13 abnormalities in multiple myeloma: a high incidence of 11q13/CCND1 and 16q23/MAF. Int J Hematol 2008;87:260–265.
105 Terpos E, Cibeira MT, Blade J, Ludwig H: Management of complications in multiple myeloma. Semin Hematol 2009;46:176–189.
106 Kyle RA, Yee GC, Somerfield MR, et al: American society of clinical oncology 2007 clinical practice guideline update on the role of bisphosphonates in multiple myeloma. J Clin Oncol 2007;25: 2464–2472.
107 Muszytowski M, Nowak J, Wojnicz M, et al: Treatment of multiple myeloma associated anemia with human recombinant erythropoietin in a hemodialysis patient. Pol Arch Med Wewn 1995;93: 77–79.
108 Bourne WM, Kyle RA, Brubaker RF, Greipp PR: Incidence of corneal crystals in the monoclonal gammopathies. Am J Ophthalmol 1989;107: 192–193.
109 Steuhl KP, Knorr M, Rohrbach JM, et al: Paraproteinemic corneal deposits in plasma cell myeloma. Am J Ophthalmol 1991;111:312–318.
110 Cherry PM, Kraft S, McGowan H, et al: Corneal and conjunctival deposits in monoclonal gammopathy. Can J Ophthalmol 1983;18:143–149.
111 Klintworth GK, Bredehoeft SJ, Reed JW: Analysis of corneal crystalline deposits in multiple myeloma. Am J Ophthalmol 1978;86:303–313.
112 Perry HD, Donnenfeld ED, Font RL: Intraepithelial corneal immunoglobulin crystals in IgG-kappa multiple myeloma. Cornea 1993;12:448–450.
113 Kleta R, Blair SC, Bernardini I, et al: Keratopathy of multiple myeloma masquerading as corneal crystals of ocular cystinosis. Mayo Clin Proc 2004;79: 410–412.
114 Knapp AJ, Gartner S, Henkind P: Multiple myeloma and its ocular manifestations. Surv Ophthalmol 1987;31:343–351.
115 Sasaki H, Kato T, Murakami A, et al: A case of monoclonal gammopathy with corneal stroma deposits. Nippon Ganka Gakkai Zasshi 2006;110: 307–311.
116 Kato T, Nakayasu K, Omata Y, et al: Corneal deposits as an alerting sign of monoclonal gammopathy: a case report. Cornea 1999;18:734–738.
117 Garibaldi DC, Gottsch J, de la Cruz Z, et al: Immunotactoid keratopathy: a clinicopathologic case report and a review of reports of corneal involvement in systemic paraproteinemias. Surv Ophthalmol 2005;50:61–80.
118 Ormerod LD, Collin HB, Dohlman CH, et al: Paraproteinemic crystalline keratopathy. Ophthalmology 1988;95:202–212.
119 Hawkins AS, Stein RM, Gaines BI, Deutsch TA: Ocular deposition of copper associated with multiple myeloma. Am J Ophthalmol 2001;131: 257–259.

120 Martin NF, Kincaid MC, Stark WJ, et al: Ocular copper deposition associated with pulmonary carcinoma, IgG monoclonal gammopathy and hypercupremia. A clinicopathologic correlation. Ophthalmology 1983;90:110–116.
121 Kyle RA: 'Benign' monoclonal gammopathy. A misnomer? JAMA 1984;251:1849–1854.
122 Gorovoy MS, Stern GA, Hood CI, Allen C: Intrastromal noninflammatory bacterial colonization of a corneal graft. Arch Ophthalmol 1983;101: 1749–1752.
123 Dunn S, Maguen E, Rao NA: Noninflammatory bacterial infiltration of a corneal graft. Cornea 1985; 4:189–193.
124 Khater TT, Jones DB, Wilhelmus KR: Infectious crystalline keratopathy caused by gram-negative bacteria. Am J Ophthalmol 1997;124:19–23.
125 Matoba AY, O'Brien TP, Wilhelmus KR, Jones DB: Infectious crystalline keratopathy due to Streptococcus pneumoniae. Possible association with serotype. Ophthalmology 1994;101:1000–1004.
126 Connell B, Armstrong M, Tullo A: A case of recurrent infectious crystalline keratopathy secondary to Haemophilus influenzae. Eye 2007;21:427–428.
127 Hu FR: Infectious crystalline keratopathy caused by mycobacterium fortuitum and oseudomonas aeruginosa. Am J Ophthalmol 1990;109:738–739.
128 Wilhelmus KR, Robinson NM: Infectious crystalline keratopathy caused by candida albicans. Am J Ophthalmol 1991;112:322–325.
129 Tu EY, Joslin CE, Nijm LM, et al: Polymicrobial keratitis: Acanthamoeba and infectious crystalline keratopathy. Am J Ophthalmol 2009;148:13–19, e2.
130 Meisler DM, Langston RH, Naab TJ, et al: Infectious crystalline keratopathy. Am J Ophthalmol 1984;97: 337–343.
131 Sridhar MS, Sharma S, Garg P, Rao GN: Epithelial infectious crystalline keratopathy. Am J Ophthalmol 2001;131:255–257.
132 Samples JR, Baumgartner SD, Binder PS: Infectious crystalline keratopathy: an electron microscope analysis. Cornea 1985;4:118–126.
133 Ainbinder DJ, Parmley VC, Mader TH, Nelson ML: Infectious crystalline keratopathy caused by candida guilliermondii. Am J Ophthalmol 1998;125: 723–725.
134 Sharma N, Vajpayee RB, Pushker N, Vajpayee M: Infectious crystalline keratopathy. CLAO J 2000;26: 40–43.
135 James CB, McDonnell PJ, Falcon MG: Infectious crystalline keratopathy. Br J Ophthalmol 1988;72: 628–630.
136 Rauber A: Observations on the idioblasts of dieffenbachia. J Toxicol Clin Toxicol 1985;23:79–90.
137 Chiou AG, Cadez R, Bohnke M: Diagnosis of dieffenbachia induced corneal injury by confocal microscopy. Br J Ophthalmol 1997;81:168–169.
138 Matysik A: Harmful impact of diffenbachia sap on the anterior segment of the eye. Klin Oczna 1996;98: 311–314.
139 Egerer I: Ocular involvement due to the juice of dieffenbachia plants (author's transl). Klin Monatsbl Augenheilkd 1977;170:128–130.
140 Tierney DW: Ocular chrysiasis. J Am Optom Assoc 1988;59:960–962.
141 Grubb BR, Matthews DO, Bentley PJ: Ocular chrysiasis: accumulation of gold in the rabbit eye. Curr Eye Res 1986;5:891–893.
142 Kincaid MC, Green WR, Hoover RE, Schenck PH: Ocular chrysiasis. Arch Ophthalmol 1982;100: 1791–1794.
143 Lopez JD, del Castillo JM, Lopez CD, Sanchez JG: Confocal microscopy in ocular chrysiasis. Cornea 2003;22:573–575.
144 Singh AD, Puri P, Amos RS: Deposition of gold in ocular structures, although known, is rare. A case of ocular chrysiasis in a patient of rheumatoid arthritis on gold treatment is presented. Eye 2004;18: 443–444.
145 Phua YS, Patel DV, McGhee CN: In vivo confocal microstructural analysis of corneal endothelial changes in a patient on long-term chlorpromazine therapy. Graefes Arch Clin Exp Ophthalmol 2005; 243:721–723.
146 Webber SK, Domniz Y, Sutton GL, et al: Corneal deposition after high-dose chlorpromazine hydrochloride therapy. Cornea 2001;20:217–219.
147 Razeghinejad MR, Nowroozzadeh MH, Zamani M, Amini N: In vivo observations of chlorpromazine ocular deposits in a patient on long-term chlorpromazine therapy. Clin Experiment Ophthalmol 2008; 36:560–563.
148 Coyle JT: Hydroxychloroquine retinopathy. Ophthalmology 2001;108:243–244.
149 Lyons JS, Severns ML: Detection of early hydroxychloroquine retinal toxicity enhanced by ring ratio analysis of multifocal electroretinography. Am J Ophthalmol 2007;143:801–809.
150 Slowik C, Somodi S, von Gruben C, et al: Detection of morphological corneal changes caused by chloroquine therapy using confocal in vivo microscopy. Ophthalmologe 1997;94:147–151.
151 Dosso A, Rungger-Brandle E: In vivo confocal microscopy in hydroxychloroquine-induced keratopathy. Graefes Arch Clin Exp Ophthalmol 2007; 245:318–320.
152 Mavrikakis I, Sfikakis PP, Mavrikakis E, et al: The incidence of irreversible retinal toxicity in patients treated with hydroxychloroquine: a reappraisal. Ophthalmology 2003;110:1321–1326.

153 Sritharan M: Studies on the tissue distribution of liposome-associated clofazimine, an antileprosy drug. Methods Find Exp Clin Pharmacol 1993;15: 107–111.
154 Kaur I, Ram J, Kumar B, et al: Effect of clofazimine on eye in multibacillary leprosy. Indian J Lepr 1990; 62:87–90.
155 Font RL, Sobol W, Matoba A: Polychromatic corneal and conjunctival crystals secondary to clofazimine therapy in a leper. Ophthalmology 1989;96: 311–315.
156 Walinder PE, Gip L, Stempa M: Corneal changes in patients treated with clofazimine. Br J Ophthalmol 1976;60:526–528.

Jayne S. Weiss, MD
Chair of Department of Ophthalmology
Herbert Kaufman, Professor of Ophthalmology
Louisiana State University Health Science Center
2020 Gravier Street, New Orleans, LA 70112 (USA)
E-Mail jayneweiss@aol.com

Lisch W, Seitz B (eds): Corneal Dystrophies.
Dev Ophthalmol. Basel, Karger, 2011, vol 48, pp 97–115

Clinical and Basic Aspects of Gelatinous Drop-Like Corneal Dystrophy

Satoshi Kawasaki · Shigeru Kinoshita

Department of Ophthalmology, Kyoto Prefectural University of Medicine, Kyoto, Japan

Abstract

Gelatinous drop-like corneal dystrophy (GDLD) was first reported in 1914 as a peculiar corneal dystrophy with an autosomal recessive inheritance mode. GDLD is rare in many countries, but relatively prevalent in Japan. The typical finding of GDLD is grayish, mulberry-like, protruding subepithelial depositions with a prominent hyperfluorescence of the cornea. Histologically, GDLD corneas are characterized by subepithelial amyloid depositions that were identified as lactoferrin by amino acid sequencing analysis. In 1998, the TACSTD2 gene was identified as a causative gene for this disease through a linkage analysis and a candidate gene approach. To date, 14 reports have demonstrated 21 mutations comprised of 9 missense, 6 nonsense, and 6 frameshift mutations from 9 ethnic backgrounds. Currently, it is hypothesized that the loss of TACSTD2 gene function causes decreased epithelial barrier function, thereby facilitating tear fluid permeation into corneal tissue, the permeated lactoferrin then transforming into amyloid depositions via an unknown mechanism. For the visual rehabilitation of patients with GDLD, ophthalmologists currently employ various types of keratoplasties; however, almost all patients will experience a recurrence of the disease within a few years after such interventions. Wearing of a soft contact lens is sometimes considered as an alternative treatment for GDLD.

Gelatinous drop-like corneal dystrophy (GDLD, MIM No. 204870) was first described in 1914 as a rare, inheritable corneal dystrophy characterized by subepithelial amyloid depositions [1]. This disease has notable features compared to other inherited corneal dystrophies. Firstly, there is a wide range of clinical appearances of GDLD, while the range of clinical appearances of most of the other inheritable corneal dystrophies is limited. Also, while the amyloid depositions of other corneal amyloidoses are derived from mutated protein of their causative genes, those of GDLD are not derived from the protein products of its causative gene but from other proteins. In addition, this disease is much more prevalent in Japan than in other countries, possibly due to the high frequency of consanguineous marriage in Japan. Here, we describe the clinical and basic aspects of GDLD.

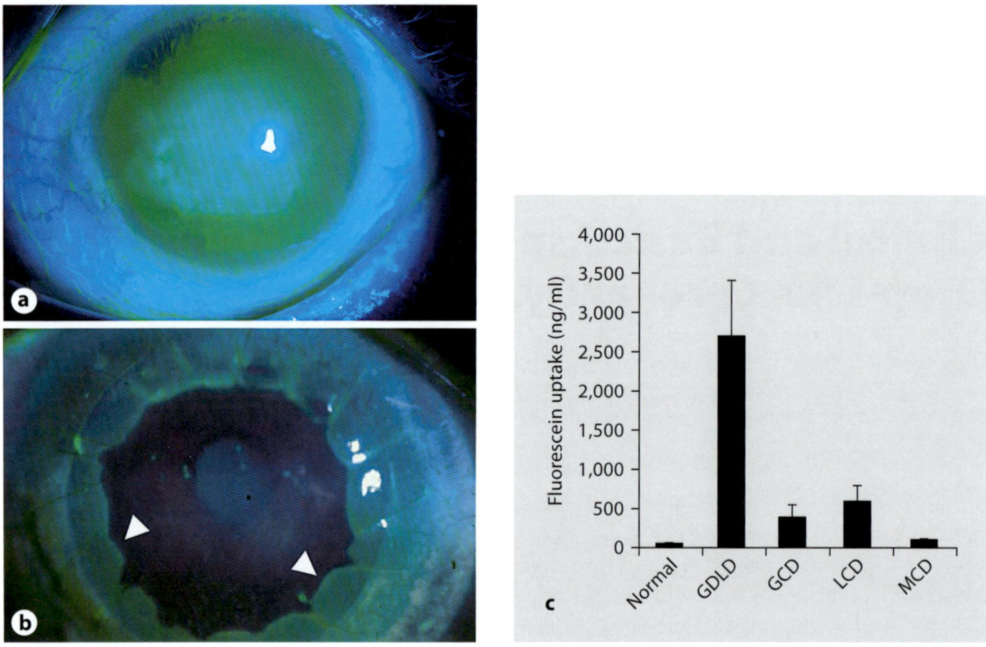

Fig. 1. **a** A slit lamp microscope photograph of the hyperfluorescence of the cornea in a GDLD patient. Note that the hyperfluorescent region covers almost the entire cornea as well as the limbus. **b** A slit lamp microscope photograph demonstrating a GDLD cornea that underwent keratoplasty. The triangle represents the boundary between the host corneal epithelium and the donated corneal epithelium. Note that the host corneal epithelium demonstrates hyperfluorescence while that of the donated cornea does not. **c** A bar graph demonstrating fluorescein uptake among several corneal dystrophies. GCD = Granular corneal dystrophy; LCD = lattice corneal dystrophy type I; MCD = macular corneal dystrophy. Note that fluorescein uptake is significantly increased in the GDLD cornea.

Clinical Features

General Clinical Properties

Clinical symptoms of GDLD include significant decrease in vision, photophobia, irritation, redness, and tearing. This disease is rare in many countries, but predominant in Japan. The prevalence rate of this disease was estimated as 1 in 31,546 from the frequency of parental consanguinity [2, 3], and the inheritance mode of this disease is autosomal recessive. The typical finding of this disease is grayish, mulberry-like, protruding subepithelial depositions which are mainly located at the central region of bilateral corneas. The onset of this disease characteristically occurs between the first and second decade of the patient's life. Typically, the corneal lesions will gradually increase in size and number and coalesce with age [4, 5]. Neovascularization of the subepithelial and superficial stroma frequently becomes evident in the very later stages [6]. One of the most prominent clinical features of this disease is increased fluorescence permeation of the corneal epithelium (fig. 1) [7], and it is almost always observed in this disease.

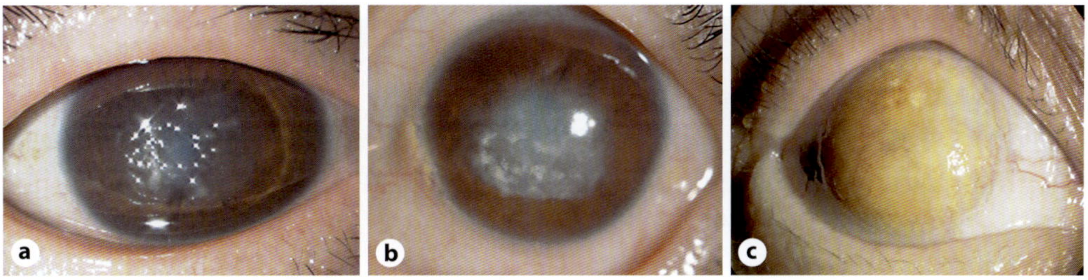

Fig. 2. An array of slit lamp microscope photographs demonstrating phenotypic variations of GDLD corneas: mulberry type (**a**), band keratopathy type (**b**), and kumquat-like type (**c**).

Subclassification of GDLD

It has been reported that GDLD can be clinically divided into 4 subtypes by the appearance of corneal opacities [8]. These subtypes include the mulberry type (fig. 2a), the band keratopathy type (fig. 2b), the kumquat-like type (fig. 2c), and stromal opacity type. Among them, the 2 predominant clinical forms are the mulberry type and the band keratopathy type. As to the causative factors of such phenotypic variations, the varying sites of mutation were initially thought to be the reason; however, in that report the authors found no apparent difference among these 4 subtypes. In addition, there have been reports demonstrating the existence of GDLD patients who have one phenotype in one eye yet a different phenotype in their other eye [8, 9]. Moreover, a previous report demonstrated the existence of a patient with band keratopathy that changed into GDLD over a 2-year period [10]. Furthermore, a previous report demonstrated the existence of a GDLD family with 1 member suffering from 1 GDLD subtype and another member suffering from a different GDLD subtype [11]. There has also been a report demonstrating a phenotypic transition from the band keratopathy type to the typical mulberry type GDLD 2 years after lamellar keratoplasty [12]. These observations strongly support the notion that the critical factors for determining the GDLD phenotype may hinge on environmental factors rather than genetic backgrounds. Some unknown factors may interfere with the process of amyloid formation, thereby affecting the phenotype of GDLD corneas. It is also speculated that such phenotypic variations are reflective of differences in the stage of GDLD. The mulberry type and the band keratopathy type tend to occur in the early to intermediate stage, while the kumquat-like type tends to occur in the very later stage.

Differential Diagnosis

The diagnosis of GDLD is frequently difficult and even cornea experts may make a misdiagnosis because its clinical appearance is not always typical but sometimes widely varied as mentioned above. The band keratopathy type GDLD exhibits an appearance that is easily confused with 'true' band keratopathy, and hence it is very probable that most patients with this GDLD subtype are misdiagnosed as such common corneal dystrophy. In addition, this GDLD subtype is sometimes misdiagnosed as spheroid degeneration, a rare corneal dystrophy which mainly affects men who work outdoors [13]. The kumquat-like type GDLD may sometimes be misdiagnosed as lipid degeneration of the cornea from the appearance of its corneal opacity. Gelatino-lattice corneal dystrophy, a rare form of TGFBI-related corneal dystrophy [14], also clinically resembles GDLD. Secondary amyloidosis sometimes presents an appearance that is confused with that of GDLD.

For the accurate diagnosis of GDLD differentially from these confusing diseases, the most important clinical manifestation appears to be hyperfluorescence of the cornea, as GDLD corneas always present a prominent finding while the diseases that GDLD is confused with do not. However, there are some misleading conditions which demonstrate a hyperfluorescence of the cornea at a level comparable to that of GDLD. One such example is drug toxicity. GDLD patients are sometimes misdiagnosed with drug toxicity, especially when they do not present apparent amyloid depositions in their corneas. However, there are various ways to discriminate between drug toxicity and GDLD. Superficial punctate keratopathy is generally found in drug toxicity but not in GDLD. In addition, in GDLD, the hyperfluorescent area not only covers the whole cornea but also extends to some areas of the limbus, while the limbus is not involved in drug toxicity. Moreover, cases of drug toxicity frequently involve the administration of multiple drugs, while those of GDLD normally do not.

For the discrimination of GDLD from the gelatino-lattice corneal dystrophy, mutation analysis of the TACSTD2 and TGFBI genes is valuable. Most secondary amyloidosis patients present the amyloid depositions in one eye while GDLD normally affects both eyes. In addition, eyelash adherence to the area of the amyloid depositions is frequently found in patients with this disease, and hence that finding is of great diagnostic value.

Examination

Routine examinations such as slit lamp biomicroscopy, visual acuity testing, and tonometry are not sufficient for the diagnosis of GDLD. For an accurate diagnosis of this disease differentially from the above-mentioned confusing diseases, the most reliable and valuable examination is undoubtedly the mutation analysis of the TACSTD2 gene. If the detected mutation is one of which was previously reported (table 1) [15] or one that may lead to potentially pathological protein alteration, the diagnosis will almost assuredly be that of GDLD. Therefore, the molecular diagnosis should be performed as thoroughly as possible (Appendix). However, and quite unfortunately, this type of examination is not available in most hospitals, even in advanced countries.

Another important examination is the above-mentioned fluorescent permeation test. This test is easily performed in a standard clinical setting, with minimal invasion for the patient, and thus should be performed prior to performing the molecular diagnosis. When the fluorescent dye is applied to a conjunctival sac of patients with this disease, the dye will immediately permeate into the corneal tissue of GDLD, even

Table 1. A list of mutations of the TACSTD2 gene that have been reported to date

Nucleotide change	Amino acid change	Original description	Ethnic origin	References
c.2T>G	p.Met1Arg	M1R	India	22
c.198C>A	p.Cys66X	C66X	Iran	15
c.250A>T	p.Lys84X	K84X	Japan	30
c.322T>C	p.Cys108Arg	C108R	Japan	30
c.341T>G	p.Phe114Cys	F114C	Iran	15
c.352C>T	p.Gln118X	Q118X	Japan, China	11, 21, 24, 26, 27, 29, 31
c.352C>G	p.Gln118Glu	Q118E	India	22
c.355T>A	p.Cys119Ser	C119S	Tunisia	22
c.493_494insCCACCGCC	p.Gly165AlafsX15	9-bp ins	India	22
c.509C>A	p.Ser170X	S170X	Japan	21
c.519dupC	p.Ala174ArgfsX43	520insC	Estonia	32
c.551A>G	p.Tyr184Cys	Y184C	China	27
c.557T>C	p.Leu186Pro	L186P	Japan, Iran	15, 29
c.564delC	p.Lys189SerfsX82	870delC	Europe	22
c.581T>A	p.Val194Glu	V194E	India	22
c.619C>T	p.Gln207X	Q270X	Japan	21
c.632delA	p.Gln211ArgfsX60	632delA	Japan	21
c.653delA	p.ASP218ValfsX53	c.653delA	Turkey	28
c.679G>A	p.Glu227Lys	E227K	Iran	15
c.772_783delATC TATTACCTGinsT	p.Ile258X	772 to 783del(ATCTAT TACCTG) + 772insT	Vietnam	31
c.811delA	p.Lys271SerfsX26	1117delA	Tunisia	22

Notational conventions for the nucleotide change and amino acid change follow the guidelines for mutation nomenclature proposed by the Human Genome Variation Society.

though corneas of GDLD patients appear to be normal (fig. 1). This particular observation is always observed in both eyes of virtually all GDLD patients. However, it should be noted that the hyperfluorescence of the cornea is not limited to GDLD but is also observed in various conditions with corneal epithelial damage, including drug toxicity, dry eye, or atopic or vernal keratoconjunctivitis [16].

Genetics and Molecular Biology of Gelatinous Drop-Like Corneal Dystrophy

Identification of the Causative Gene for Gelatinous Drop-Like Corneal Dystrophy

When investigators searched for the responsible gene for GDLD, the TGFBI gene, a causative gene for various types of corneal epithelial-stromal dystrophies [17], was first examined; however, no pathological mutations were found in any of the patients with this disease [18]. Mutation analysis of the lactoferrin gene was also performed, but no pathological mutations were found in this gene [19]. In 1998, Tsujikawa et al. [20] performed a linkage analysis of 10 consanguineous Japanese families with a total of 13 affected members and found genotype-phenotype linkage with a maximum LOD score of 9.8 at the D1S2741 microsatellite marker on the short arm of chromosome 1. They also performed haplotype analysis and further defined the disease-associated locus within 2.6 cM (approximately corresponding to 2.6×10^6 bp) between the markers D1S2890 and D1S2801 [20]. Using 3 additional markers, they further narrowed the probable range to a 400-kb critical region between the markers D1S2648 and D1S2752 [21]. Subsequently, they isolated cosmid and BAC clones covering this 400-kb critical region and determined nearly its entire sequence by the shotgun cloning method. In that region, only 1 known gene was located. They performed a candidate gene approach for this gene and found 4 different mutations in the TACSTD2 gene (alternatively named as M1S1 or TROP2) in 26 patients of 20 Japanese GDLD families [21]. The 4 mutations include p.Gln118X, p.Gln211ArgfsX60, p.Gln207X, and p.Ser170X (originally designated as Q118X, 632delA, Q207X, and S170X, respectively). All of these are nonsense or frameshift mutations, thus producing truncated protein lacking a computationally predicted transmembrane domain located near the C-terminal region of this gene. Subsequently, Ren et al. [22] also performed linkage analyses of 8 unrelated GDLD families from different ethnic backgrounds (Indian, European, Tunisian) other than Japanese. They found that in 7 of those families the disease locus fell to a 16-cM region at the short arm of chromosome 1, which includes the TACSTD2 gene. They also performed mutation analysis of the TACSTD2 gene and identified 7 novel mutations in those families. The 1 remaining GDLD family was found to have no mutation in the TACSTD2 gene, suggesting the existence of other genes responsible for the occurrence of GDLD as reported in other studies [23–26].

From the same sets of patients as above, Tsujikawa et al. [20] also found linkage disequilibrium between the microsatellite marker D1S220 and the p.Gln118X

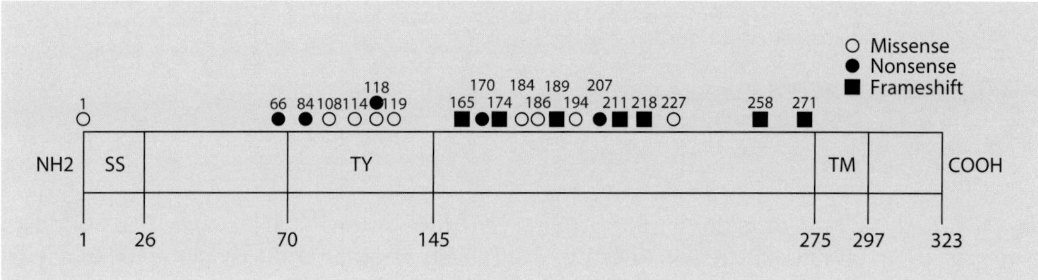

Fig. 3. Schematic representation of the distribution of TACSTD2 mutations and the domain structure of the TACSTD2 protein. SS = Signal sequence; TY = thyroglobulin-like domain; TM = transmembrane domain. All mutations are depicted with amino acid numbers and their effects on protein change such as missense (○), nonsense (●), and frameshift (■).

mutation, suggesting that GDLD patients bearing this nonsense mutation all descended from the same ancestor in whom the founder mutation occurred. Interestingly, the p.Gln118X mutation was also found in a Chinese GDLD patient [27]. Possibly, that patient's mutation descended from the putative founder mutation in common with all of the Japanese GDLD patients bearing the p.Gln118X mutation.

Mutation Analysis

After the determination of the TACSTD2 gene as the gene responsible for this disease, a large number of mutation studies have been made on GDLD patients in different countries with different ethnic backgrounds. At the time of writing, there have been 13 reports demonstrating 21 mutations comprised of 14 substitution, 4 deletion, and 2 insertion mutations, as well as 1 delins (a condition where insertion occurs in a deleted region) mutation, causing 9 missense, 6 nonsense, and 6 frameshift protein alterations in patients from 9 ethnic backgrounds including Japanese, Indian, Chinese, Iranian, Estonian, Turkish, Tunisian, Vietnamese, and European (table 1; fig. 3) [11, 12, 21–24, 27–33].

In spite of such allelic heterogeneity, most of the patients are homozygous and share only 1 mutation at both alleles, indicating that most GDLD patients were born to parents who are closely related. Actually, parents of GDLD patients demonstrate a frequency of consanguineous marriage of 43%, much higher than the frequency of 6.8% found in the general population [23]. Some of the parents who are not consanguineous may have the same TACSTD2 mutation in 1 of their alleles, especially when their birthplaces are close to each other. Consanguineous marriages may also be an important factor for the reason why GDLD frequently occurs in the Japanese population. In Japan, interfamily marriage (i.e. to a cousin) had historically been more common than in Western countries and is still currently permitted by law. This social tradition may have facilitated the occurrence of GDLD in this country. The fact that

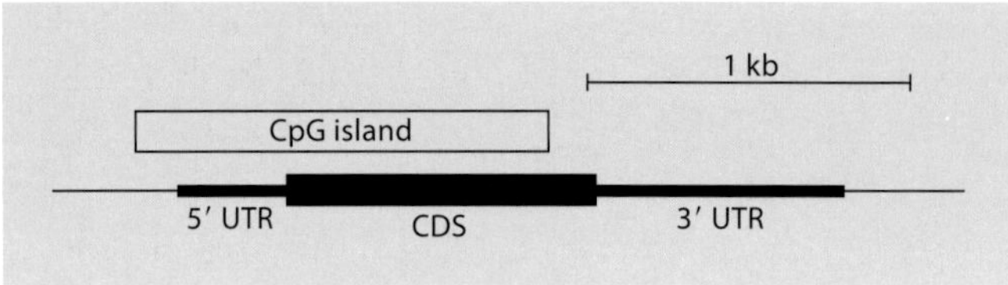

Fig. 4. Schematic representation of the genomic structure of the TACSTD2 gene. CDS = Coding sequence; UTR = untranslated region. The CpG island covers a portion of the promoter region as well as the 5′ UTR and more than 3/4 of the CDS of the TACSTD2 gene.

Japan is a relatively heavily populated country with an advanced national healthcare system may also be a factor as to why GDLD is more frequently seen in this country. Since the trend of consanguineous marriage is on the decrease in Japan, especially in recent years [34], it is expected that the incidence of GDLD in this country will gradually begin to mirror that decrease in the near future.

Although the number is small, the GDLD of some patients was reportedly caused by compound heterozygous mutations [21, 27, 30, 31], a rare condition where one mutation occurs in one allele and another mutation occurs in another allele. Such complicated situations suggest that most of the sporadic cases of GDLD may be born to nonconsanguineous normal parents, both bearing different TACSTD2 mutations from each other. With the recent decrease in the frequency of consanguineous marriage in Japan, the sporadic cases should eventually begin to outnumber the familial cases in this country.

Genomic Structure of the TACSTD2 Gene

TACSTD2 is a single-exon gene comprised of a central coding region flanked by 5′ and 3′ untranslated regions (fig. 4). There are 22 single nucleotide polymorphisms in this gene, which potentially affect the expression and function of this gene. The promoter region of this gene contains several consensus sequences which are potentially recognized by various transcription factors. Of note, TATA and GC box consensus sequences, which are respectively known as binding motifs for the transcription-initiating complex and ubiquitous transcription factor Sp1, are found at multiple sites upstream of the translation start site. The transcription start site for this gene has not been experimentally determined. However, expressed sequence tag analysis done for various purposes in research areas unrelated to ophthalmology imply the existence of 2 major transcription start sites located downstream of the 5′ end of a reference sequence (NM_002353, Refseq) of the TACSTD2 gene. Interestingly, more than half of the region of this gene, including its promoter, is significantly CpG rich (fig. 4). The so-called CpG island [35, 36] is often found in the upstream regions of many genes and is believed to be important for the regulation of gene expression. In general, when the cytosine residues of the CpG island are methylated, expression of the gene will

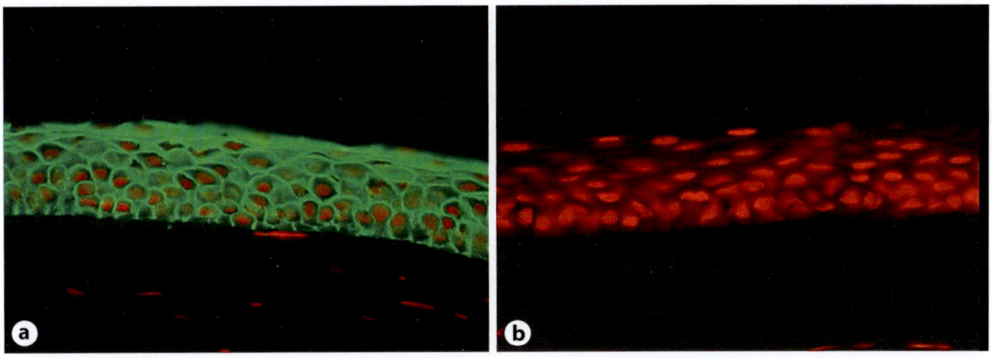

Fig. 5. A photograph representing immunolocalization of TACSTD2 protein in normal and GDLD corneal epithelia. Green signals = Immunoreaction to TACSTD2 protein; red signals = nuclei stained by propidium iodide. The TACSTD2 protein is localized at the cell-to-cell borders of almost all epithelial layers in normal cornea (**a**) but virtually completely absent in GDLD cornea (**b**).

be downregulated. Therefore, the existence of the CpG island in the TACSTD2 gene implies the potential epigenetic regulation for the expression of this gene. Resolution of these issues would appear to be fundamental in order to obtain a thorough understanding of the nature of the TACSTD2 gene; however, at the time of writing, virtually no experimental data have been presented that pertain to these issues.

Expression and Functions of the TACSTD2 Gene

In a study conducted in 1999, Northern blot analysis revealed that organs such as the cornea, placenta, lung, kidney, pancreas, and prostate express mRNA of the TACSTD2 gene [21]. TACSTD2 protein is thought to be a single-pass type I membrane protein consisting of 323 amino acids with a molecular weight of 35,709 Da. In that study, the authors also reported that forcedly expressed TACSTD2 protein was subcellularly localized to cytoplasm in COS-7 and HeLa cells. However, a subsequent study from another group has shown discrepant data that this protein was localized at the cell-to-cell border when forcedly expressed in CHO cells [31]. Human corneal tissue expresses this protein at the plasma membrane of all epithelial layers (our unpublished data, fig. 5). The protein functions of the TACSTD2 gene have yet to be fully elucidated, yet as one may imagine from the name 'tumor-associated calcium signal transducer 2', the gene is thought to be involved in cancer biology. In fact, there have been several reports regarding the relationship between this gene and cancers [37–39]. In these studies, the TACSTD2 gene has been reported to be highly expressed in many kinds of cancer cells and is thought to play an important role in the maintenance or facilitation of cancer cells. Interestingly, the epithelial cell adhesion molecule, the gene most homologous to the TACSTD2 gene, has also been reported to be highly expressed in many kinds of cancers [40–42] and has currently become an attractive and popular target for tumor therapy. In fact, there have been several clinical trials utilizing monoclonal [43, 44] or bispecific antibodies [45, 46] and vaccination strategies [47] against this gene with varying degrees of success. Other than its relevance to cancer, the TACSTD2 gene was reported to be coupled with calcium signaling from the fact that the intercellular calcium concentration was dramatically changed when OvCa-432 cells were treated with anti-TACSTD2 antibody [48]. In addition, it has been demonstrated that in GDLD corneas, tight-junction-related proteins such as ZO-1, occludin, and claudin 1 are eliminated from the most apical side of the lateral junctions of the superficial cells [49], strongly suggesting that TACSTD2 protein may play an important role in the formation or maturation of the tight junction.

Computationally Predicted Attributes of TACSTD2 Protein

Several biological, chemical, and physical attributes can be computationally predicted for the TACSTD2 gene. SOSUI, a transmembrane domain prediction software [50], has shown that there are 2 potential transmembrane domains in this gene, and another transmembrane domain prediction software, one that employs the hidden Markov model algorithm (TMHMM) [51], also demonstrated nearly the same results. SignalP, a software used for predicting a signal sequence that is characteristic of secreted or membrane proteins [52], predicted the existence of a signal peptide and cleavage site at the N-terminus of TACSTD2 protein (fig. 3). Since the predicted signal peptide almost matches one of the transmembrane domains, the TACSTD2 gene supposedly has only 1 transmembrane domain near its C-terminus (fig. 3). PROSITE, a protein motif database [53], predicts that TACSTD2 protein has a thyroglobulin type 1 domain profile at its 70- to 145-amino acid region (fig. 3). PSORT, a software used for predicting the subcellular localization of proteins [54], implies that this protein is localized to the plasma membrane with a statistical certainty of 0.46, to the endoplasmic reticulum with a statistical certainty of 0.38, and to lysosomes with a statistical certainty of 0.20. The homologous gene for TACSTD2 can be determined by use of a homology search software such as BLAST [55]. By use of such software, it was discovered that the best-aligned gene is epithelial cell adhesion molecule, with a 50% similarity to the TACSTD2 gene.

Pathogenicity of TACSTD2 Mutations

Nearly two thirds of the mutations of the TACSTD2 gene that have so far been reported in GDLD patients are nonsense or frameshift mutations (deletion, insertion, and delins) which potentially lead to truncation of the TACSTD2 protein. It can easily be predicted that such alterations may lead to a change in the subcellular localization of this protein because all of these truncated TACSTD2 proteins lack the putative C-terminal hydrophobic transmembrane domain, and hence lose the capacity to be localized at the plasma membrane.

However, there have been some reports showing the existence in patients of GDLD caused by missense mutations of the TACSTD2 gene. Of such mutations, p.Met1Arg [22] is thought to be apparently pathological because this mutation will alter the start codon methionine to arginine, and hence disrupt the translation initiation site where the ribosome apparatus will recognize and start translation. Therefore, in this case, the ribosome machinery will pass over the mutated translation initiation site, and hence its downstream ATG triplet may be recognized and work as an alternative translation initiation site. However, translation initiation generally requires not only the ATG triplet sequence but also a consensus sequence around the ATG triplet. The so-called 'Kozak' sequence is known to be the sequence, and this special sequence supposedly has the power to make the decision regarding translation strength [56, 57]. The Kozak sequence of the authentic translation initiation site of the TACSTD2 gene (–6 CCCACCAUGG +4) is nearly identical to the typical Kozak consensus sequence (–6 GCCA/GCCAUGG +4), suggesting that the translation strength of this gene is very high. As no potential Kozak sequences are found either upstream or downstream of the authentic Kozak sequence of the TACSTD2 gene, it is highly theorized that virtually no protein will be produced from the TACSTD2 gene bearing the p.Met1Arg mutation, although mRNA may be transcribed from this mutated TACSTD2 gene as high as the wild-type TACSTD2 gene.

Strictly speaking, it is still unclear as to whether other missense mutations are truly pathological or not. However, acceptable theoretical explanations have been given for some of those mutations. Frequently given explanations are that (1) the mutation causes amino acid transition with change in chemical properties such as from polar amino acid to nonpolar amino acid, or that (2) the mutation is found in affected family members but not found in unaffected family members in an affected pedigree (phenotype-genotype cosegregation), or that (3) the mutation is located on the putatively functional domains, thereby disrupting the protein function, or that (4) the mutation is found in GDLD patients but not found in normal volunteers, or that (5) the mutation is located at regions that are highly conserved among orthologous genes in animals and/or among paralogous genes in humans. A change in some specific amino acid is sometimes thought to be pathological. For example, mutations causing amino acid transition from cysteine to another amino acid [31] or a certain amino acid to cysteine [28] are expected to produce considerable impacts on the function of this gene, possibly through the disruption or the creation of the disulfide bond between 2 cysteine residues. However, since most single nucleotide polymorphisms in most genes are thought to be potentially nonpathological even if they carry changes in amino acid, such explanations are kinds of desk theories and they should be validated in the future through experiments.

Pathophysiology of the Gelatinous Drop-Like Corneal Dystrophy Cornea

Histology

Histologically, the GDLD cornea is characterized by subepithelial amyloid depositions, which can be recognized as an amorphous substance stained in red by hematoxylin-eosin staining. The amyloid depositions are also specifically stained in red by Congo-red staining (fig. 6a), and those Congo-red-stained amyloid depositions demonstrate yellow-green birefringence when observed by a polarized microscope (fig. 6b). The corneal epithelium over the subepithelial amyloid depositions becomes thinner with a reduced number of epithelial layers and an absence of the Bowman's membrane. However, the corneal epithelium over the regions without amyloid depositions appears to be normal with normal thickness and the normal number of epithelial layers, as well as an intact Bowman's membrane [58]. Scanning electron microscopy also demonstrated that a larger number of desquamating cells were observed in the superficial cells of the GDLD cornea than in the normal cornea (fig. 6c) [7]. The scanning electron microscopy analysis also demonstrated that some of the apical intercellular junctions are loosened in the GDLD cornea (fig. 6d), while the normal cornea did not show such a prominent change [7]. Moreover, examination by electron microscopy indicated that horseradish peroxidase, a molecular tracer with a molecular weight of 40 kDa, permeated through the corneal epithelial barrier of a GDLD patient, while normal corneal epithelium did not allow this tracer to permeate into this tissue (fig. 6e) [59]. These observations, along with the clinically observed hyperfluorescence of the cornea in GDLD, are the main reason for our current hypothesis that epithelial barrier function may be severely damaged in the GDLD cornea.

Causative Protein for the Amyloid Depositions of the Gelatinous Drop-Like Corneal Dystrophy Cornea

In a study by Klintworth et al. [60], it was reported that a 78-kDa protein band exists in samples taken from GDLD corneas, whereas control samples did not show this protein band. In that study, amino acid sequencing analysis disclosed that the protein band was derived from lactoferrin. By Western blot analysis, the authors confirmed that the 78-kDa protein band is actually lactoferrin. Using an immunohistochemistry technique, they also found that the amyloid depositions in the GDLD cornea were really reacted with an antibody against lactoferrin. From these observations, they initially supposed that mutation of the lactoferrin gene may be responsible for the occurrence of GDLD; however, a subsequent study by that group showed that no mutations were found in the lactoferrin gene of GDLD patients [19].

Since an earlier study has demonstrated that apolipoproteins A and J exist in amyloid depositions [61], it is possible that not a single protein but, in fact, multiple proteins may participate in the formation of amyloid depositions of GDLD.

Pathogenesis of Gelatinous Drop-Like Corneal Dystrophy

Without question, the homozygous mutation of the TACSTD2 gene, which results in the loss of function of this gene, is definitely a primary reason for the occurrence

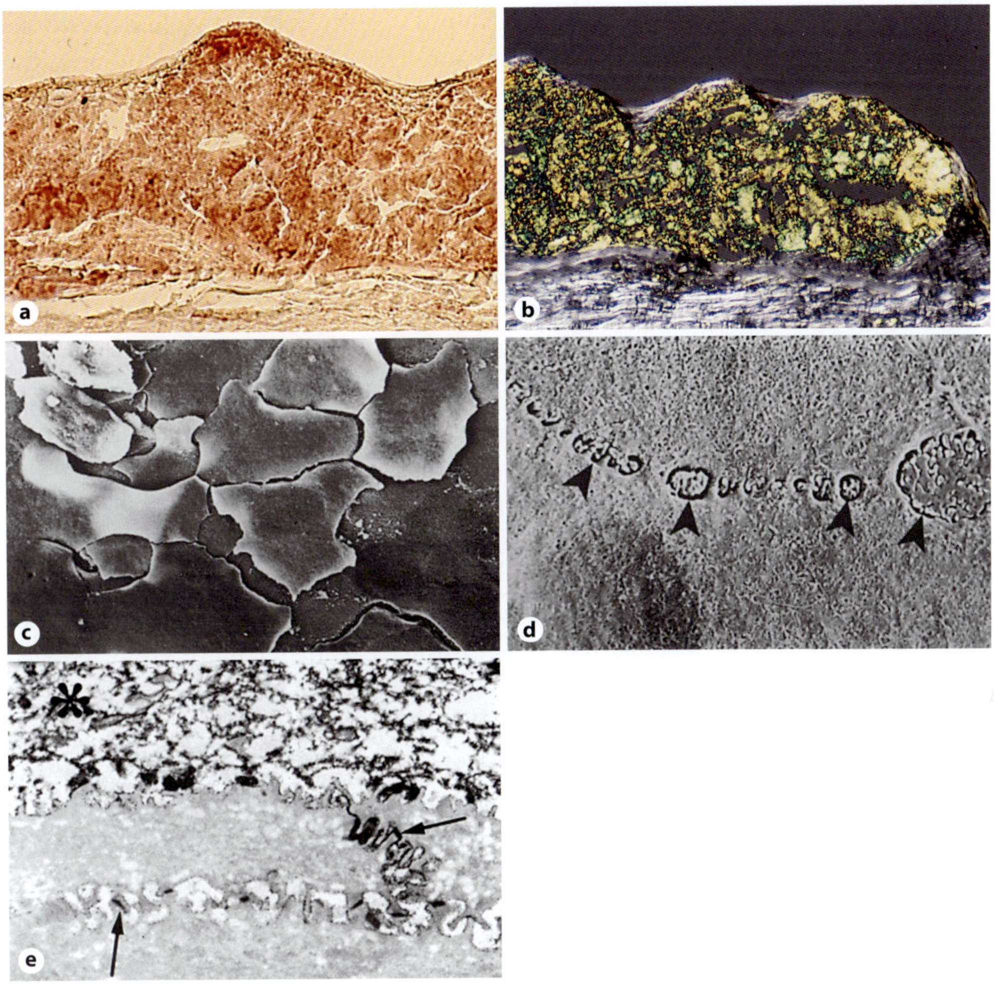

Fig. 6. An array of photographs showing histological examinations of GDLD cornea by congo red staining (**a**), Congo red staining by a polarized microscope (**b**), scanning electron microscopy (**c, d**), transmission electron microscopy. Arrows indicate permeated HRP residing intracellularly (**e**).

of GDLD. The decreased epithelial barrier function via the reduced expression of the epithelial tight-junction-related proteins seems to be the subsequent pathological event. The pathological event that next follows appears to be permeation of tear fluid through the loosened epithelial barrier function. Finally, the permeated tear lactoferrin may form amyloid depositions. This is our current concept for the pathogenesis of GDLD. However, there are still many aspects of this disease that have yet to be elucidated, issues such as why the loss of function of the TACSTD2 gene causes the reduced expression of the tight-junction-related proteins. In addition, it has yet to be explained why the lactoferrin protein, which is normally water-soluble in the tear fluid, transforms into water-insoluble amyloid depositions when the protein permeates into corneal tissue. These 2 questions should be at the forefront of any future investigation aiming to formulate a complete understanding of this disease.

Treatment Strategies for Gelatinous Drop-Like Corneal Dystrophy

Surgical Strategies

Various types of treatments have been reported for GDLD. Currently, penetrating keratoplasty, deep lamellar keratoplasty, lamellar keratoplasty, and superficial keratectomy are the standard surgical procedures for this disease. However, almost all patients will develop recurrence within a few years after such interventions and repeated keratoplasties are frequently required for GDLD patients [62]. Therefore, less invasive procedures should be considered, especially for the patient's first surgical treatment. Complications associated with these treatments include glaucoma, infection, and rejection of the corneal graft. However, and although the reason for this phenomenon is currently unknown, there seems to be a tendency that steroid-induced glaucoma frequently occurs, and is much more severe, in GDLD. It is speculated that amyloid depositions may also exist in the trabecular meshwork of GDLD patients, and hence give those patients an inclination towards increased intraocular pressure. Since the loss of function of the TACSTD2 gene in the corneal epithelium is currently believed to be a primary reason for the pathogenesis of this disease, allogeneic transplantation of normal limbal tissue is sometimes considered [63]. This procedure completely replaces the patient's limbal epithelial cells with the donated ones. Thereafter, the transplanted corneal epithelial cells, which potentially have normal TACSTD2 gene function, will be regenerated from the transplanted limbal tissue, totally cover the patient's cornea, and result in epithelial barrier function that is nearly normal. Since the epithelial cells are more inclined towards allogeneic rejection than are corneal endothelial cells [64–66], high-dose immunosuppressive agents are frequently administrated to promote longevity of the transplanted limbal epithelial cells.

Contact Lens Wear

One promising alternative treatment for GDLD is soft contact lens wear. Although the underlying mechanism of how/why this treatment provides a beneficial effect on GDLD is currently unknown, we get the impression that the wearing of a soft contact lens actually retards the progression of this disease. The wearing of a soft contact lens may possibly decrease the local turnover of tear fluid around the corneal surface, thereby decreasing the permeation of tear fluid into corneal tissue. Alternatively, wearing of the lens may possibly enhance the physical integrity of the corneal epithelium, probably by protecting the epithelium from the shear stress that occurs at the time of blinking. Although it can be omitted in early GDLD cases, pretreatment by

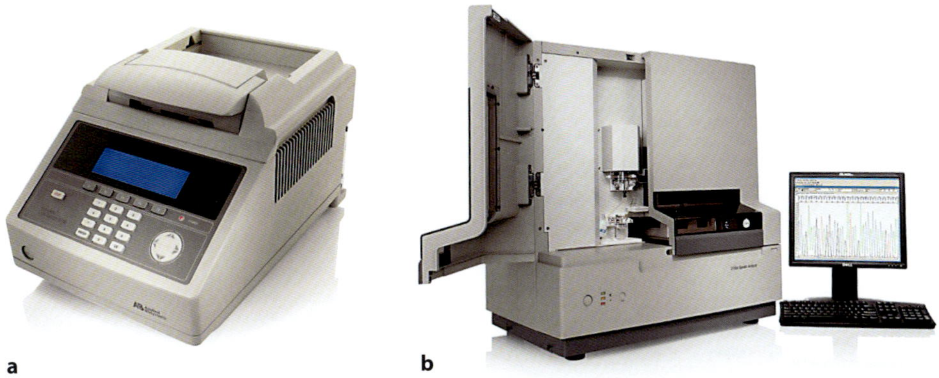

a b

Fig. A1. An array of photographs representing equipments used in the molecular diagnosis of GDLD: thermal cycler (GeneAmp® PCR System 9700, Applied Biosystems) (**a**) and automated sequencer (3130xl Genetic Analyzer, Applied Biosystems) (**b**).

excimer laser ablation using a smoothing technique [67] is preferable so that corneal protrusions are removed to alleviate foreign body sensation or pain during wearing of the soft contact lens.

Appendix: Laboratory System for the Molecular Diagnosis of Gelatinous Drop-Like Corneal Dystrophy

Since molecular diagnosis is frequently unavailable in most hospitals, researchers who intend to make an accurate diagnosis for patients with GDLD will often need to self-construct a system for molecular diagnosis. The minimum set of required equipment includes a thermal cycler (fig. A1a), an automated sequencer (fig. A1b), and a microcentrifuge. After setting up the required equipment, the first step is to extract genomic DNA from the patient's peripheral blood. This is most easily accomplished by use of a commercial column-based DNA extraction kit that is available from numerous companies. The second step is to amplify the extracted DNA using a primer pair which should surround the entire coding sequence of the TACSTD2 gene. Since the GC content of the coding sequence of this gene is relatively high (ca. 67.5%), it is beneficial to add 10% dimethyl sulfoxide into the PCR buffer, although it is highly dependent upon the experimental conditions. In our experimental condition, the 'touchdown' thermal condition [68] was found to be more preferable than the normal thermal condition. Tables A1 and A2 represent our current regimen for the PCR amplification of the TACSTD2 gene. The PCR product should be checked by electrophoresis on an agarose gel. After this confirmation, the PCR product should be purified by use of a commercially available purification kit to remove unreacted primers and dNTP because they will significantly reduce the efficiency of the subsequent sequencing reaction. There are many types of kits on the market specifically designed for this purpose. The most convenient purification kit may be a mixture of exonuclease I and shrimp alkaline phosphatase which cleaves the primer and dNTP, respectively. Then, the purified/treated PCR product can be used as a template for the sequencing reaction by the use of a commercial sequencing kit. The product of the sequencing reaction should be purified by a gel filtration (e.g. G50) or a simple ethanol precipitation. Then, the purified prod-

Table A1. The PCR parameters currently used for mutation analysis of the TACSTD2 gene

Forward primer	CCTGCAGACCATCCCAGAC
Reverse primer	CAGGAAGCGTGACTCACTTG
Enzyme	ExTaq
Buffer	1 × Vogelstein buffer
dNTP	1.25 mM
Mg^{2+}	3.9 mM
Additive	10% dimethyl sulfoxide
Thermal condition	touchdown

The Vogelstein buffer contains 67 mM Tris-HCl, 16.6 mM $(NH_4)_2SO_4$, 0.07% 2-mercaptoethanol and 0.067 mM EDTA.

Table A2. The thermal profile of touchdown PCR for the amplification of TACSTD2 gene

Step	Temperature/duration	Purpose	Repeats
1	94°C/3 min	denature	1
2	94°C/30 s, 70°C/1 min	amplification	3
3	94°C/30 s, 68°C/1 min	amplification	3
4	94°C/30 s, 66°C/1 min	amplification	3
5	94°C/30 s, 64°C/1 min	amplification	3
6	94°C/30 s, 62°C/1 min	amplification	3
7	94°C/30 s, 60°C/1 min	amplification	3
8	94°C/30 s, 58°C/30 s, 72°C/1 min	amplification	3
9	94°C/30 s, 55°C/30 s, 72°C/1 min	amplification	30
10	72°C/5 min	elongation	1

uct is ready for electrophoresis on an automated fluorescence sequencer. The obtained sequence data should then be analyzed by alignment software. Web-based free alignment software [e.g. BLAST (http://blast.ncbi.nlm.nih.gov/Blast.cgi) or Clustal W2 (http://www.ebi.ac.uk/Tools/clustalw2/)] is often sufficient for this purpose; however, well-designed, intelligent alignment software programs (e.g. Variant Reporter, Applied Biosystems) are available from some companies and are quite helpful for easy identification of gene mutations.

Acknowledgements

The authors wish to thank Dr. Tsutomu Inatomi for his insightful advice for the clinical section of this chapter. The authors also thank John Bush and Hideki Fukuoka for their excellent help in the preparation of this chapter, and Dr. Andrew Quantock for providing us with the excellent photographs used in this chapter.

References

1 Nakaizumi G: A rare case of corneal dystrophy. Acta Soc Ophthalmol Jpn 1914;18:949–950.

2 Fukjiki K, Kanai A, Nakajima A: Gelatinous drop-like corneal dystrophy in Japanese population (abstract). 7th Int Congr Hum Genet 1986, Berlin, pp 248–249.

3 Kawano H, Fujiki K, Kanai A, Nakajima A: Prevalence of gelatinous drop-like corneal dystrophy in Japan. Atarashii Ganka 1992;9:1879–1882.

4 Weber FL, Babel J: Gelatinous drop-like dystrophy. A form of primary corneal amyloidosis. Arch Ophthalmol 1980;98:144–148.

5 Mondino BJ, Rabb MF, Sugar J, Sundar Raj CV, Brown SI: Primary familial amyloidosis of the cornea. Am J Ophthalmol 1981;92:732–736.

6 Fujita S, Sameshima M, Hirashima S, Nakao K: Light and electron microscopic study of gelatinous drop-like corneal dystrophy with deeper stromal involvement. Nippon Ganka Gakkai Zasshi 1988;92: 1744–1757.

7 Kinoshita S, Nishida K, Dota A, Inatomi T, Koizumi N, Elliott A, Lewis D, Quantock A, Fullwood N: Epithelial barrier function and ultrastructure of gelatinous drop-like corneal dystrophy. Cornea 2000;19:551–555.

8 Ide T, Nishida K, Maeda N, Tsujikawa M, Yamamoto S, Watanabe H, Tano Y: A spectrum of clinical manifestations of gelatinous drop-like corneal dystrophy in Japan. Am J Ophthalmol 2004;137: 1081–1084.

9 Akiya S, Takahashi H, Furukawa H, Hamada T, Sugahara S, Suzuki T, Ninomiya H, Yoshimura M, Shimazaki J, Tsubota K, et al: A case of one eye with gelatinous drop-like corneal dystrophy and the other eye with band-shaped spheroidal corneal degeneration. Ophthalmologica 1995;209: 96–100.

10 Kanai A, Kaufman HE: Electron microscopic studies of primary band-shaped keratopathy and gelatinous, drop-like corneal dystrophy in two brothers. Ann Ophthalmol 1982;14:535–539.

11 Yoshida S, Kumano Y, Yoshida A, Numa S, Yabe N, Hisatomi T, Nishida T, Ishibashi T, Matsui T: Two brothers with gelatinous drop-like dystrophy at different stages of the disease: role of mutational analysis. Am J Ophthalmol 2002;133:830–832.

12 Ha NT, Fujiki K, Hotta Y, Nakayasu K, Kanai A: Q118X mutation of M1S1 gene caused gelatinous drop-like corneal dystrophy: the P501T of BIGH3 gene found in a family with gelatinous drop-like corneal dystrophy. Am J Ophthalmol 2000;130: 119–120.

13 Smolin G: Corneal dystrophies and degenerations; in Smolin G, Thoft RA (eds): The Cornea, ed 3. Boston, Little, Brown and Co, 1994, pp 507–508.

14 Nakamura T, Nishida K, Dota A, Adachi W, Yamamoto S, Maeda N, Okada M, Kinoshita S: Gelatino-lattice corneal dystrophy: clinical features and mutational analysis. Am J Ophthalmol 2000; 129:665–666.

15 Weiss JS, Moller HU, Lisch W, Kinoshita S, Aldave AJ, Belin MW, Kivela T, Busin M, Munier FL, Seitz B, Sutphin J, Bredrup C, Mannis MJ, Rapuano CJ, Van Rij G, Kim EK, Klintworth GK: The IC3D classification of the corneal dystrophies. Cornea 2008; 27(suppl 2):S1–S83.

16 Kinoshita S, Adachi W, Sotozono C, Nishida K, Yokoi N, Quantock AJ, Okubo K: Characteristics of the human ocular surface epithelium. Prog Retin Eye Res 2001;20:639–673.

17 Munier FL, Korvatska E, Djemai A, Le Paslier D, Zografos L, Pescia G, Schorderet DF: Kerato-epithelin mutations in four 5q31-linked corneal dystrophies. Nat Genet 1997;15:247–251.

18 Dota A, Nishida K, Honma Y, Adachi W, Kawasaki S, Quantock AJ, Kinoshita S: Gelatinous drop-like corneal dystrophy is not one of the beta ig-h3-mutated corneal amyloidoses. Am J Ophthalmol 1998;126:832–833.

19 Klintworth GK, Sommer JR, Obrian G, Han L, Ahmed MN, Qumsiyeh MB, Lin PY, Basti S, Reddy MK, Kanai A, Hotta Y, Sugar J, Kumaramanickavel G, Munier F, Schorderet DF, El Matri L, Iwata F, Kaiser-Kupfer M, Nagata M, Nakayasu K, Hejtmancik JF, Teng CT: Familial subepithelial corneal amyloidosis (gelatinous drop-like corneal dystrophy): exclusion of linkage to lactoferrin gene. Mol Vis 1998;4:31.

20 Tsujikawa M, Kurahashi H, Tanaka T, Okada M, Yamamoto S, Maeda N, Watanabe H, Inoue Y, Kiridoshi A, Matsumoto K, Ohashi Y, Kinoshita S, Shimomura Y, Nakamura Y, Tano Y: Homozygosity mapping of a gene responsible for gelatinous drop-like corneal dystrophy to chromosome 1p. Am J Hum Genet 1998;63:1073–1077.

21 Tsujikawa M, Kurahashi H, Tanaka T, Nishida K, Shimomura Y, Tano Y, Nakamura Y: Identification of the gene responsible for gelatinous drop-like corneal dystrophy. Nat Genet 1999;21:420–423.

22 Ren Z, Lin PY, Klintworth GK, Iwata F, Munier FL, Schorderet DF, El Matri L, Theendakara V, Basti S, Reddy M, Hejtmancik JF: Allelic and locus heterogeneity in autosomal recessive gelatinous drop-like corneal dystrophy. Hum Genet 2002;110:568–577.

23 Fujiki K, Nakayasu K, Kanai A: Corneal dystrophies in Japan. J Hum Genet 2001;46:431–435.

24 Yajima T, Fujiki K, Murakami A, Nakayasu K: Gelatinous drop-like corneal dystrophy: mutation analysis of membrane component, chromosome 1, surface marker 1. Nippon Ganka Gakkai Zasshi 2002;106:265–272.
25 Akhtar S, Bron AJ, Qin X, Creer RC, Guggenheim JA, Meek KM: Gelatinous drop-like corneal dystrophy in a child with developmental delay: clinicopathological features and exclusion of the M1S1 gene. Eye 2005;19:198–204.
26 Alavi A, Elahi E, Amoli FA, Tehrani MH: Exclusion of TACSTD2 in an Iranian GDLD pedigree. Mol Vis 2007;13:1441–1445.
27 Tian X, Fujiki K, Li Q, Murakami A, Xie P, Kanai A, Wang W, Liu Z: Compound heterozygous mutations of M1S1 gene in gelatinous droplike corneal dystrophy. Am J Ophthalmol 2004;137: 567–569.
28 Alavi A, Elahi E, Tehrani MH, Amoli FA, Javadi MA, Rafati N, Chiani M, Banihosseini SS, Bayat B, Kalhor R, Amini SS: Four mutations (three novel, one founder) in TACSTD2 among Iranian GDLD patients. Invest Ophthalmol Vis Sci 2007;48: 4490–4497.
29 Markoff A, Bogdanova N, Uhlig CE, Groppe M, Horst J, Kennerknecht I: A novel TACSTD2 gene mutation in a Turkish family with a gelatinous drop-like corneal dystrophy. Mol Vis 2006;12: 1473–1476.
30 Taniguchi Y, Tsujikawa M, Hibino S, Tsujikawa K, Tanaka T, Kiridoushi A, Tano Y: A novel missense mutation in a Japanese patient with gelatinous droplike corneal dystrophy. Am J Ophthalmol 2005;139: 186–188.
31 Murakami A, Kimura S, Fujiki K, Fujimaki T, Kanai A: Mutations in the membrane component, chromosome 1, surface marker 1 (M1S1) gene in gelatinous drop-like corneal dystrophy. Jpn J Ophthalmol 2004;48:317–320.
32 Ha NT, Chau HM, Cung le X, Thanh TK, Fujiki K, Murakami A, Kanai A: A novel mutation of M1S1 gene found in a Vietnamese patient with gelatinous droplike corneal dystrophy. Am J Ophthalmol 2003; 135:390–393.
33 Tasa G, Kals J, Muru K, Juronen E, Piirsoo A, Veromann S, Janes S, Mikelsaar AV, Lang A: A novel mutation in the M1S1 gene responsible for gelatinous droplike corneal dystrophy. Invest Ophthalmol Vis Sci 2001;42:2762–2764.
34 Imaizumi Y: A recent survey of consanguineous marriages in Japan. Clin Genet 1986;30:230–233.
35 Gardiner-Garden M, Frommer M: CpG islands in vertebrate genomes. J Mol Biol 1987;196:261–282.
36 Takai D, Jones PA: The CpG island searcher: a new WWW resource. In Silico Biol 2003;3:235–240.
37 Fong D, Spizzo G, Gostner JM, Gastl G, Moser P, Krammel C, Gerhard S, Rasse M, Laimer K: TROP2: a novel prognostic marker in squamous cell carcinoma of the oral cavity. Mod Pathol 2008;21: 186–191.
38 Fong D, Moser P, Krammel C, Gostner JM, Margreiter R, Mitterer M, Gastl G, Spizzo G: High expression of TROP2 correlates with poor prognosis in pancreatic cancer. Br J Cancer 2008;99: 1290–1295.
39 Muhlmann G, Spizzo G, Gostner J, Zitt M, Maier H, Moser P, Gastl G, Zitt M, Muller HM, Margreiter R, Ofner D, Fong D: TROP2 expression as prognostic marker for gastric carcinoma. J Clin Pathol 2009;62: 152–158.
40 Spizzo G, Went P, Dirnhofer S, Obrist P, Moch H, Baeuerle PA, Mueller-Holzner E, Marth C, Gastl G, Zeimet AG: Overexpression of epithelial cell adhesion molecule (Ep-CAM) is an independent prognostic marker for reduced survival of patients with epithelial ovarian cancer. Gynecol Oncol 2006;103: 483–488.
41 Gastl G, Spizzo G, Obrist P, Dunser M, Mikuz G: Ep-CAM overexpression in breast cancer as a predictor of survival. Lancet 2000;356:1981–1982.
42 Litvinov SV, van Driel W, van Rhijn CM, Bakker HA, van Krieken H, Fleuren GJ, Warnaar SO: Expression of Ep-CAM in cervical squamous epithelia correlates with an increased proliferation and the disappearance of markers for terminal differentiation. Am J Pathol 1996;148:865–875.
43 Sears HF, Atkinson B, Mattis J, Ernst C, Herlyn D, Steplewski Z, Hayry P, Koprowski H: Phase-I clinical trial of monoclonal antibody in treatment of gastrointestinal tumours. Lancet 1982;i:762–765.
44 Sears HF, Herlyn D, Steplewski Z, Koprowski H: Effects of monoclonal antibody immunotherapy on patients with gastrointestinal adenocarcinoma. J Biol Response Mod 1984;3:138–150.
45 Gronau SS, Schmitt M, Thess B, Reinhardt P, Wiesneth M, Schmitt A, Riechelmann H: Trifunctional bispecific antibody-induced tumor cell lysis of squamous cell carcinomas of the upper aerodigestive tract. Head Neck 2005;27:376–382.
46 Riesenberg R, Buchner A, Pohla H, Lindhofer H: Lysis of prostate carcinoma cells by trifunctional bispecific antibodies (alpha EpCAM x alpha CD3). J Histochem Cytochem 2001;49:911–917.
47 Neidhart J, Allen KO, Barlow DL, Carpenter M, Shaw DR, Triozzi PL, Conry RM: Immunization of colorectal cancer patients with recombinant baculovirus-derived KSA (Ep-CAM) formulated with monophosphoryl lipid A in liposomal emulsion, with and without granulocyte-macrophage colony-stimulating factor. Vaccine 2004;22: 773–780.

48 Ripani E, Sacchetti A, Corda D, Alberti S: Human Trop-2 is a tumor-associated calcium signal transducer. Int J Cancer 1998;76:671–676.
49 Takaoka M, Nakamura T, Ban Y, Kinoshita S: Phenotypic investigation of cell junction-related proteins in gelatinous drop-like corneal dystrophy. Invest Ophthalmol Vis Sci 2007;48:1095–1101.
50 Hirokawa T, Boon-Chieng S, Mitaku S: SOSUI: classification and secondary structure prediction system for membrane proteins. Bioinformatics 1998;14: 378–379.
51 Bagos PG, Liakopoulos TD, Hamodrakas SJ: Algorithms for incorporating prior topological information in HMMs: application to transmembrane proteins. BMC Bioinformatics 2006;7:189.
52 Bendtsen JD, Nielsen H, von Heijne G, Brunak S: Improved prediction of signal peptides: SignalP 3.0. J Mol Biol 2004;340:783–795.
53 Hulo N, Bairoch A, Bulliard V, Cerutti L, Cuche BA, de Castro E, Lachaize C, Langendijk-Genevaux PS, Sigrist CJ: The 20 years of PROSITE. Nucleic Acids Res 2008;36:D245–D249.
54 Nakai K, Horton P: PSORT: a program for detecting sorting signals in proteins and predicting their subcellular localization. Trends Biochem Sci 1999;24: 34–36.
55 Altschul SF, Gish W, Miller W, Myers EW, Lipman DJ: Basic local alignment search tool. J Mol Biol 1990;215:403–410.
56 Kozak M: At least six nucleotides preceding the AUG initiator codon enhance translation in mammalian cells. J Mol Biol 1987;196:947–950.
57 Kozak M: Recognition of AUG and alternative initiator codons is augmented by G in position +4 but is not generally affected by the nucleotides in positions +5 and +6. EMBO J 1997;16:2482–2492.
58 Ohnishi Y, Shinoda Y, Ishibashi T, Taniguchi Y: The origin of amyloid in gelatinous drop-like corneal dystrophy. Curr Eye Res 1982;2:225–231.
59 Quantock AJ, Nishida K, Kinoshita S: Histopathology of recurrent gelatinous drop-like corneal dystrophy. Cornea 1998;17:215–221.
60 Klintworth GK, Valnickova Z, Kielar RA, Baratz KH, Campbell RJ, Enghild JJ: Familial subepithelial corneal amyloidosis – A lactoferrin-related amyloidosis. Invest Ophthalmol Vis Sci 1997;38:2756–2763.
61 Nishida K, Quantock AJ, Dota A, Choi-Miura NH, Kinoshita S: Apolipoproteins J and E co-localise with amyloid in gelatinous drop-like and lattice type I corneal dystrophies. Br J Ophthalmol 1999;83: 1178–1182.
62 Ohzono S, Ogawa K, Kinoshita S, Moriyama H, Manabe R: Recurrence of corneal dystrophy following keratoplasty. Rinsho Ganka 1984;38:747–749.
63 Shimazaki J, Shimmura S, Tsubota K: Limbal stem cell transplantation for the treatment of subepithelial amyloidosis of the cornea (gelatinous drop-like dystrophy). Cornea 2002;21:177–180.
64 Yamada J, Streilein JW: Induction of anterior chamber-associated immune deviation by corneal allografts placed in the anterior chamber. Invest Ophthalmol Vis Sci 1997;38:2833–2843.
65 Hori J, Joyce N, Streilein JW: Epithelium-deficient corneal allografts display immune privilege beneath the kidney capsule. Invest Ophthalmol Vis Sci 2000; 41:443–452.
66 Yao YF, Inoue Y, Miyazaki D, Shimomura Y, Ohashi Y, Tano Y: Ocular resurfacing and alloepithelial rejection in a murine keratoepithelioplasty model. Invest Ophthalmol Vis Sci 1995;36:2623–2633.
67 Hersh PS, Burnstein Y, Carr J, Etwaru G, Mayers M: Excimer laser phototherapeutic keratectomy. Surgical strategies and clinical outcomes. Ophthalmology 1996;103:1210–1222.
68 Don RH, Cox PT, Wainwright BJ, Baker K, Mattick JS: 'Touchdown' PCR to circumvent spurious priming during gene amplification. Nucleic Acids Res 1991;19:4008.

Satoshi Kawasaki, MD, PhD
465 Kajii-cho, Hirokoji-agaru
Kawaramachi-dori
Kamigyo-ku, Kyoto 602–0841 (Japan)
Tel. +81 75 251 5578, E-Mail bluenova@koto.kpu-m.ac.jp

Lisch W, Seitz B (eds): Corneal Dystrophies.
Dev Ophthalmol. Basel, Karger, 2011, vol 48, pp 116–153

Stage-Related Therapy of Corneal Dystrophies

Berthold Seitz[a] · Walter Lisch[b]

[a]Department of Ophthalmology, University of Saarland, Homburg/Saar, and [b]Department of Ophthalmology, City Hospital of Hanau, Hanau, Germany

Abstract

Corneal dystrophies typically result in a gradual bilateral loss of vision in a primary 'white eye' – often in conjunction with epithelial defects in later stages. Treatment of corneal dystrophies needs to be stage-related. To ensure a stage-related therapeutic approach, an adequate classification based on clinical, histopathological and genetic knowledge is indispensable. In principle, topical medications, contact lenses and various microsurgical approaches are applicable. In case of predominantly superficial dystrophies of the epithelium, basal membrane and/or Bowman's layer (map-dot-fingerprint, Meesmann, Lisch, Reis-Bücklers, Thiel-Behnke), recurrent epithelial defects may complicate the clinical picture. If conservative therapy with gels/ointments, application of therapeutic contact lenses and/or conventional corneal abrasion are not successful, phototherapeutic keratectomy (PTK) using a 193-nm excimer laser is the method of choice today. PTK can be repeated several times, thus postponing corneal transplantation (lamellar or even penetrating) for a long time. Three major goals may be achieved by PTK depending on the diagnosis: (1) to remove superficial opacities; (2) to regularize the surface and treat irregular astigmatism, and (3) to improve the adherence of the epithelium. In dystrophies with depositions predominantly in the stroma (e.g. granular, lattice, macular, recurrence on the graft), PTK may be a reasonable alternative to anterior lamellar or penetrating keratoplasty (PKP) depending on the exact localization of the lesions. Besides exact determination of the depth of depositions using a slit lamp, a preoperative topography analysis is indispensable. The therapy of endothelial dystrophies depends on diagnosis and age: Fuchs endothelial corneal dystrophy will need corneal transplantation (e.g. when visual acuity drops below 0.4). In contrast, transplantation will only be very rarely necessary in posterior polymorphous corneal dystrophy, but the intraocular pressure has to be checked frequently. Especially in elderly patients with reduced compliance, posterior lamellar keratoplasty – preferably in the form of Descemet stripping automated endothelial keratoplasty – may be performed instead of PKP. In case of congenital hereditary endothelial dystrophy, the best time point of PKP has to be determined with regard to amblyopia (surgery too late) and inadequate follow-up (surgery too early) together with parents and pediatric ophthalmologists on an individual basis. In conclusion, for stage-related therapy of corneal dystrophies, besides contact lenses, PTK and PKP, various techniques of lamellar keratoplasties represent an indispensable enrichment of our corneal microsurgical spectrum today.

Corneal dystrophies typically result in a gradual bilateral loss of vision in a primary 'white eye' – often in conjunction with epithelial defects in later stages. Treatment of corneal dystrophies needs to be stage-related. To ensure a stage-related therapeutic approach, an adequate classification based on clinical, histopathological and genetic knowledge is indispensable. In principle, topical medications, contact lenses and microsurgical interventions are applicable.

Over the past decades, there has been a shift in treatment of these conditions from corneal transplantation (penetrating keratoplasty – PKP) to excimer laser-assisted keratectomy, typically referred to today as phototherapeutic keratectomy (PTK), for visual restoration. PTK using the 193-nm excimer laser can produce significant visual improvement in these patients, and corneal transplantation or repeat transplantation can be delayed or even avoided. In addition, lamellar keratoplasty techniques [anterior lamellar keratoplasty (ALKP) and posterior lamellar keratoplasty (PLKP)] are widely discussed today.

Phototherapeutic Keratectomy Using an Excimer Laser

In case of predominantly superficial dystrophies of the epithelium, basal membrane and/or Bowman's layer (map-dot-fingerprint, Meesmann, Lisch, Reis-Bücklers, Thiel-Behnke), recurrent epithelial defects may complicate the clinical picture. If conservative therapy with gels/ointments, application of therapeutic contact lenses and/or conventional corneal abrasion are not successful, PTK using a 193-nm excimer laser is the method of choice today [1]. PTK can be repeated several times, thus postponing corneal transplantation (lamellar or even penetrating) for a long time. Three major goals may be achieved by PTK depending on the diagnosis: (1) to remove superficial opacities; (2) to regularize the surface and treat irregular astigmatism, and (3) to improve the adherence of the epithelium. These three goals may apply to variable degrees in a given pathology (fig. 1) [2].

In dystrophies with depositions predominantly in the stroma (e.g. granular, lattice, macular, recurrence on the graft), PTK may be a reasonable alternative to anterior lamellar keratoplasty or PKP depending on the exact localization of the lesions. Besides exact determination of the depth of depositions using a slit lamp, a preoperative topography analysis is indispensable. In principle, prominent lesions have a good, whereas localized lesions with stromal thinning have a limited prognosis.

Patient Counseling

The efficacy of PTK seems to be related to several factors, including (1) the nature of the corneal disorder; (2) the patient's subjective complaints; (3) the preoperative refractive error; (4) the treatment strategy, and (5) the tissue ablation properties

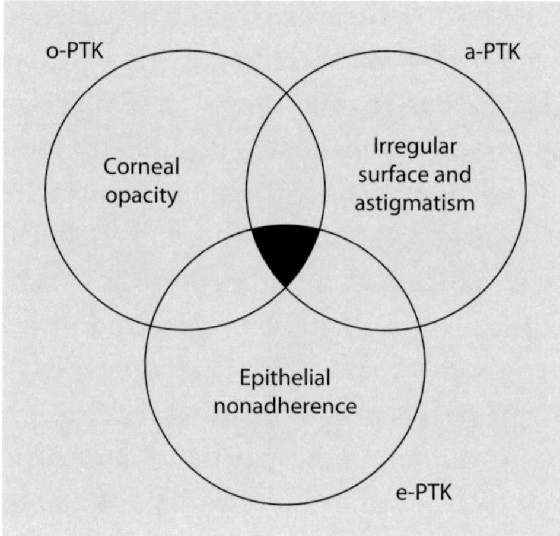

Fig. 1. Indications for PTK: (1) corneal opacity (o-PTK); (2) irregular corneal surface and astigmatism (a-PTK), and (3) epithelial nonadherence (e-PTK). Such indications may overlap in a number of corneal disease processes and may apply to variable degrees in a given pathology (modified after Hersh and Wagoner [2]).

of the laser. Careful attention should be directed toward the specific patient complaints to better determine if PTK may be expected to achieve the desired clinical goals. Certainly, the patient should be completely informed about the diverse surgical steps. Especially, characteristic phenomena referred to as 'sight', 'sound' and 'smell' have to be discussed with each patient in advance to avoid unexpected reactions intraoperatively.

Corneal Clarity

A crystal-clear cornea is typically not the goal of a PTK for superficial corneal dystrophies. The goal is to postpone or even avoid lamellar keratoplasty or PKP. Often removal of major central opacities leads to a considerable increase in visual acuity [3]. Typically some deposits are left in the midstroma (e.g. in granular dystrophy) without major disadvantages. The dystrophy may recur early after PTK, especially in macular dystrophy [4, 5] and Reis-Bücklers dystrophy [6, 7]. In contrast, map-dot-fingerprint dystrophy [8] and granular dystrophy [9, 10] will recur later. In case of recurrence of the dystrophy, repeat PTK or PKP/ALKP may be necessary [11, 12].

Visual Acuity and Refraction

Depending on the preoperative refraction, PTK may lead to an increased best-corrected visual acuity (BCVA), despite a decrease in the uncorrected visual acuity (UCVA). This may be due to a hyperopic shift after central PTK. A BCVA of 1.0 (20/20) is not the goal. Often the patient is highly satisfied when the visual acuity increases from 0.2–0.3 to 0.6–0.8. In some cases, even a hard contact lens may be necessary to achieve good vision. The patient must be aware of this potential problem in advance and should not be confronted with this issue for the first time after PTK in case a major hyperopic shift has occurred.

Recurrent Corneal Erosion Syndrome

Corneal dystrophies (especially epithelial basement membrane dystrophy – EBMD) are often associated with recurrent corneal erosion syndrome (RCES) [13]. Conservative treatment in case of RCES may include (1) gels and ointments; (2) lubricants (to be applied especially early in the morning and late at night); (3) nonpreserved artificial tears in severe cases; (4) autologous serum [14]; (5) therapeutic contact lenses, or (6) collagen shields.

Surgical alternatives include (1) abrasion and thorough removal of the basal membrane with a hockey knife, with or without (2) anterior stromal puncture [15]. Anterior stromal puncture should not be performed in the central optical zone to avoid glare, halos and visual impairment postoperatively. After PTK, the success rate is not 100% but somewhere between 85 and 90% [16, 17]. Artificial tears and/or gels are still necessary after PTK. Especially if PTK in corneal dystrophy is performed predominantly because of the pain caused by RCES, the patient must be aware of the potential loss of UCVA after PTK.

Diagnostic Approaches for Surgical Decision Making

Microsurgeons should realize that PTK is not the treatment of choice for all anterior corneal pathologies. 'Aiming and shooting' at all corneal pathologies should be avoided to prevent dissatisfaction and frustration. The primary diagnosis does not necessarily dictate the treatment of choice, since various clinical presentations of the same disorder may suggest different therapeutic approaches (table 1). Appropriate recommendations regarding treatment of choice can be made only after analyzing the horizontal/vertical distribution and the pattern of the pathology [3] and the applicability of manual versus PTK techniques.

However, the ultimate determinant of the appropriate technique is the functional objective of the procedure. (1) Visual objectives relate to final visual acuity. In assessing a patient's needs not only is the final BCVA important but any potential adverse alteration in UCVA that may result from undesirable hyperopic shift must be taken into account. (2) Nonvisual objectives include (a) reducing pain associated with RCES, which is a very typical complication of many progressive dystrophies [13], (b) decreasing optical problems such as glare, halo, monocular diplopia or triplopia, and/or (c) clearing the visual axis for subsequent cataract surgery.

Patient Selection

Besides clearly defining the expectations of patients and recheck whether these can be achieved with PTK, the individual corneal pathology itself is most critical for surgical decision making. Contact lens tolerance should be an issue in the process of decision making before surgery. In contrast to refractive surgery or even laser PKP, the PTK procedure has to be planned on an individual basis. Therefore, it is essential that the

Table 1. Principal therapeutic options for corneal dystrophies

Conservative
Topical (artificial tears, gels, ointment; antibiotics)
Contact lenses (soft/rigid; with/without keratoplasty)
Surgical
Corneal abrasion/pannus removal
Phototherapeutic keratectomy (with/without mitomycin C)
Corneal transplantation
Penetrating keratoplasty
Conventional
Excimer laser
Femtosecond laser
Deep anterior lamellar keratoplasty
Posterior lamellar keratoplasty (DSAEK, DMEK)

DSAEK = Descemet stripping automated endothelial keratoplasty; DMEK = Descemet membrane endothelial keratoplasty.

surgeon has a close look at the cornea using a slit lamp immediately before surgery, even if he/she has seen the patient at an earlier visit.

Refractometry

Identical morphological presentations do not necessarily dictate the same treatment of choice, since functional requirements may suggest different therapeutic approaches. Reis-Bücklers corneal dystrophy (RBCD) in a myopic eye may be successfully treated with PTK. In contrast, the same pathology in a hyperopic eye may suggest only manual superficial keratectomy, at least in case the patient is contact lens intolerant. For this reason, objective and subjective refractometry measurements of both eyes are mandatory in each patient before PTK to avoid anisometropia postoperatively.

Biomicroscopy with the Slit Lamp

Pattern Assessment

In all instances of assessment of corneal dystrophies, the light of the slit lamp must NOT be dimmed. For surgical decision making, the localization of the lesion is important: (1) multifocal (regular corneal tissue in between); (2) segmental contiguous, and (3) diffuse patterns of opacifications may be distinguished. Especially in cases of EBMD, the microsurgeon has to look carefully for subtle epithelial changes. In these cases, indirect illumination and retrograde illumination with dilated pupils may be required to detect the prevalent lesions.

Horizontal Extension

Modified after Hersh and Wagoner [2], corneal pathology may be categorized into the (1) central (optically relevant); (2) paracentral, and (3) peripheral zone.

The central zone is defined as the central 3–4 mm where the dystrophy may directly (through clouding of the visual axis) or indirectly (through the induction of irregular astigmatism) diminish visual function.

The paracentral zone is defined as the midperipheral area where pathology may indirectly affect visual function by the induction of irregular astigmatism and light scattering/glare. More often, however, treatment for disorders in this region is considered for recurrent epithelial erosions or potential extension into the visual axis. PTK in this region may produce alterations in visual function due to iatrogenic changes in the contour of adjacent corneal tissue in the visual axis.

The peripheral zone has little or no direct impact on visual function. However, in case of high elevation, for example peripheral nodules of Salzmann's corneal degeneration may induce irregular astigmatism due to tear film pooling. Multifocal (mid-) peripheral nodules may even induce considerable hyperopia and irregular astigmatism due to asymmetric tear film pooling resulting in an 'optical cornea plana' [18].

Vertical Extension

To evaluate the vertical extension, first a classification of the level of the corneal surface at the site of the lesion has to be made: (1) 'plus disease' is defined as an elevated (nodular) lesion compared to the surrounding corneal surface; (2) 'zero disease' is defined as a lesion within the level of the surrounding corneal surface, and (3) 'minus disease' is defined as a depressed lesion compared to the surrounding corneal surface. In addition, the vertical extension of corneal disorders may be divided into (1) pre-Bowman's layer; (2) involving Bowman's layer, and (3) anterior stroma, and midstroma. 'Pre-Bowman's' refers to dystrophies that involve the epithelium and basement membrane, but completely spare Bowman's layer, for example EBMD (eponym: map-dot-fingerprint dystrophy) [8].

'Bowman's' refers to all pathologies incorporated into Bowman's layer with or without epithelial and epithelial basement membrane involvement, for example Reis-Bücklers or Thiel-Behnke dystrophy [1, 2]. 'Anterior stromal' refers to dystrophies that have extended beneath Bowman's layer into the anterior 100–150 μm of the cornea, for example anterior variants of granular or lattice dystrophy [3, 9, 10]. 'Stromal' refers to disorders where excision of deep stromal lamellae (>150 μm) is required to achieve a satisfactory visual outcome, for example macular dystrophy [4, 5].

Topography Analysis and Assessment of Corneal Thickness Profile

Besides keratometry, topography analysis is indispensable to reflect the corneal power map over the central and midperipheral cornea. The effects of localized or diffuse lesions on the corneal curvature are best assessed with topography analysis. Refractive powers and individual axes of 4 or more hemimeridians are rounded up

Table 2. Strategic planning and surgical techniques of excimer laser PTK

Avoid 'aiming and shooting' at all corneal pathologies to avoid dissatisfaction and frustration
Remove as much of the diseased tissue with the blade
Remove as little tissue as possible with the laser (see fig. 2)
Use the laser predominantly for smoothing
Use 'masking agents' repeatedly during one session
Consider simultaneous refractive ablation
Prevention of hyperopic shift with deep ablation
High/irregular astigmatism and superficial opacities (topography-based ablation)
Asymmetric astigmatism after PKP and recurrence of dystrophies
Recentration of the apex with medium-stage keratoconus (in case of contact lens intolerance)
Take into account potential subsequent PKP (save peripheral Bowman's layer for suture fixation)

by system-specific indices, such as surface regularity index and surface asymmetry index of the TMS topography system [19].

Ultrasound pachymetry can only supply the microsurgeon with the entire corneal thickness at one spot. In contrast, slit scanning tomography (Orbscan) or Scheimpflug analysis (Pentacam) provide a thickness profile of the cornea including full information on the anterior and posterior corneal curvature. To assess the true vertical involvement of the lesion, anterior segment optical coherence tomography may be used. Nevertheless, slit lamp examination still is the most important qualitative examination technique to plan the surgical approach.

Strategic Planning and Surgical Techniques

PTK is not necessarily the treatment of choice for all anterior corneal pathologies. While in many circumstances it represents a significant advance in our ability to excise pathology that was once difficult to remove manually, it does not always guarantee a superior result. In some situations, it may produce an even less desirable outcome than manual superficial keratectomy (table 2).

General Concepts

In each individual patient, the actual ability of the PTK procedure to accomplish the desired objective of removing the pathologic process AND regularize the surface must be ascertained. Almost invariably, any dystrophy amenable to manual resection can be removed by PTK, although the converse is not true. Generally, the more posterior the pathology extends the more likely manual keratectomy is to be technically less desirable than PTK. At Bowman's layer, disorders such as Reis-Bücklers or Thiel-Behnke dystrophy may be easily resected manually. In contrast, anterior

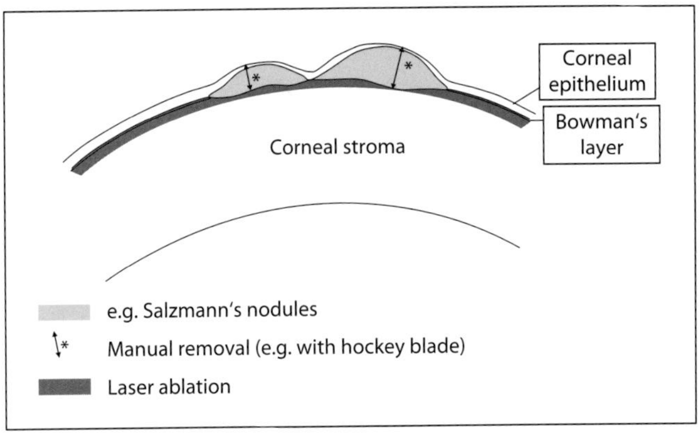

Fig. 2. Technical details: first major prominent subepithelial tissue is removed manually, e.g. with a hockey blade, before excimer laser ablation is applied to remove intrastromal opacifications and especially smoothen the surface (by use of masking fluids) [23, 24].

corneal dystrophies reaching into the stroma (e.g. granular or lattice dystrophy) are typically very difficult to remove manually with a blade but are amenable to PTK [3, 18].

In general, PTK should be performed on a 'quiet eye'. Possible confounding problems such as blepharitis and active infection must be controlled before proceeding with surgery. In addition, intraocular inflammation should be controlled. The intended effects of PTK may be threefold: (1) removal of corneal opacities; (2) treatment of irregular corneal surface and astigmatism, and (3) increase and stabilization of epithelial adherence. Such indications may overlap in a number of corneal diseases and may apply to variable degrees in a given pathology (fig. 1).

Removal of Opacities

Generally, we recommend to remove as much of the diseased tissue with the blade or hockey knife and remove as little tissue as possible with the laser. This is especially true for all 'plus diseases' which are multifocally arranged. A cleavage plane is identified between abnormal tissue and Bowman's layer or stroma using the hockey knife to raise a tissue edge. To facilitate visualization and manipulation of the abnormal tissue, the corneal surface is kept dry. Traction may be applied with a forceps to strip the abnormal material along its natural cleavage plane while the tip of a dry cellulose sponge may be used as an atraumatic dissection instrument. In the case of strong adherence, the blade may be carefully used to lyse adhesions or to scrape residual abnormal tissue. Care is taken to leave limbal stem cells intact [20, 21]. Caution should be taken to remain in the cleavage plane, thus avoiding damage to Bowman's layer that may evoke further corneal scarring and irregularities. After mechanical scraping of residual tissue remnants with the hockey knife, laser ablation is performed. This technique may be called 'subepithelial PTK' (fig. 2).

In case of regular corneal topography – which is very rarely the case – a 'transepithelial PTK' may be advisable. In this case, the epithelium will mask the irregularities

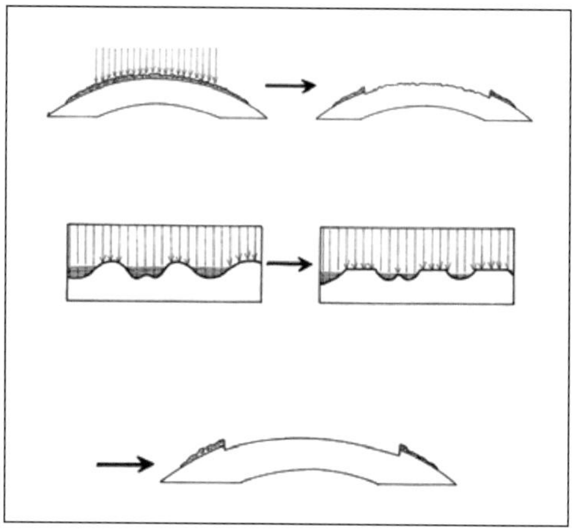

Fig. 3. Application of masking fluid to smoothen the corneal surface. Upper left/right: schematic drawing of an irregular corneal surface before/after excimer laser ablation. Note how the irregular corneal surface pattern is preserved although the corneal substance is thinned. Middle left/right: using a masking fluid to protect the 'valleys' of the corneal surface by absorbing incoming laser energy will allow smoothing of the surface as the 'peaks' of the irregular surface are removed by photoablation leaving a smooth corneal surface (bottom) (modified after Hersh and Wagoner [2]).

of the superficial stroma, acting as a biological 'masking agent' and contributing to a smoother postoperative stromal surface. However, different ablation rates in epithelium, stroma and scar tissue have to be taken into account.

Microsurgeons should be aware of the fact that corneal dystrophies typically recur after some time. Thus, removing as little tissue as possible (although the cornea may not be completely cleared) and leaving enough tissue to enable repeat PTK is mandatory. Especially in case of stromal involvement of dystrophies, corneal transplantation may be required later, if the outcome is not satisfactory for the patient. Therefore, peripheral Bowman's layer should be saved for suture fixation in case of subsequent PKP [22]. Typically, a treatment diameter of 7.0–8.0 mm with a small transition zone of around 0.5 mm is adequate.

Smoothening of Surface and Decreasing Irregular Astigmatism

It is important to note that, in general, the excimer laser will remove an equivalent amount of tissue over the entire area upon which it impinges (fig. 3). Although opacities will be removed, irregularities of the surface will be maintained because tissue is removed parallel to the surface. Therefore, during most PTK procedures it is mandatory to use so-called 'masking fluids' repeatedly during one session. Methylcellulose 1% has proven to fill in irregularities, thereby smoothing the surface to be ablated [2]. Hyaluronic acid 0.3% (e.g. Vismed®) may also be used successfully for this purpose [23]. The viscosity of these fluids is appropriate to fill in the 'valleys' of an irregular surface while leaving the 'peaks' exposed to the laser action [24]. This allows the surface to be smoothed with the laser while opacities are removed. The thickness of the masking fluid layer should be enough to smooth the valleys of the corneal surface, but not so much as to completely block the incoming laser beam. Collagen gels and other molding compounds have not been generally accepted in the community of corneal specialists.

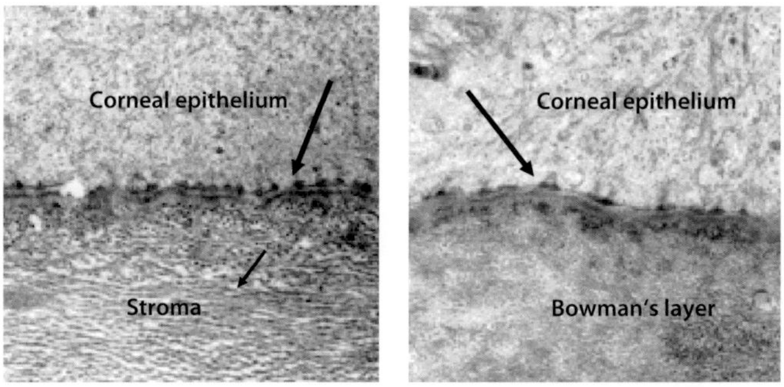

Macular dystrophy after PTK;
Density of hemidesmosomes:
5,500 ± 800/mm

Macular dystrophy - Control
Density of hemidesmosomes:
3,500 ± 900/m

Fig. 4. Increased number of hemidesmosomes may be responsible for improved epithelial adherence after excimer laser PTK in macular corneal dystrophy. Without laser ablation, 3,500 ± 900 hemidesmosomes per millimeter of basal membrane length were measured. In contrast, after PTK, 5,500 ± 800 hemidesmosomes per millimeter of basal membrane length were measured [25].

The laser procedure is interrupted at frequent intervals and the patient may be examined with the slit lamp to monitor progress of the procedure and to determine areas to be treated further. If no slit lamp is available, typically 2–3 sessions with intended ablation depths of 40–50 μm over appropriate masking fluid are sufficient to regularize the corneal stromal surface after extensive mechanical debridement.

Improvement of Epithelial Adhesion

In case of nondystrophic RCES (e.g. traumatic origin), some microsurgeons advocate transepithelial PTK with treatment scheduled in the painless interval. However, RCES in the context of progressive corneal dystrophies should preferably be treated with subepithelial PTK (= treatment of Bowman's layer after generous removal of loose and irregular epithelium).

We know from histologic and ultrastructural studies that excimer laser ablation results in a significant increase in hemidesmosomes (fig. 4) thus improving epithelial adhesion to the underlying stroma [25]. For this reason, even dystrophies, such as the map-dot-fingerprint variant, that may be removed with mechanical corneal abrasion only should better be treated with additional PTK to regularize the surface and improve epithelial adherence [8].

Combination with Mitomycin C

Combining PTK with temporary application of 0.02 mg% mitomycin C on a merocel sponge for 30–60 s after laser action may prevent scarring and recurrence of certain corneal pathologies, such as granular dystrophy type 2 and Salzmann's nodular degeneration [26]. Potential problems with this antimetabolite include: hyperopic shift, epithelial healing problems, endothelial damage in thin corneas, and irreversible keratocyte damage with (late) melting. However, corneal toxicity of mitomycin C is not well established yet.

Medical Treatment

Preoperative Treatment

Typically, nonsteroidal anti-inflammatory drugs are applied 4 times a day the day before and at the day of surgery to reduce corneal inflammatory reaction after PTK. There is no need to apply topical or systemic antibiotics before PTK. In some cases, the operative eye may require pilocarpine 1% to constrict the pupil and thereby facilitate centration of the procedure and improve visualization of the pilot beam on the cornea.

Intraoperative Treatment

Most procedures are done using only topical anesthetic drops. In case of corneal dystrophies with intended subepithelial PTK, we prefer cocaine drops to break the hemidesmosomes thus making mechanical epithelial removal easier. Intraoperatively, masking fluids may be repeatedly used to achieve a regularization of the corneal surface depending on the degree of irregularity in a given eye.

At the end of surgery, we preferably apply cyclopentolate drops and ofloxacin ointment in conjunction with a pressure patch, to be changed daily until complete epithelial closure. Other microsurgeons prefer to apply ofloxacin eyedrops and a therapeutic contact lens.

To reduce pain, we supply the patient with tramadol orally for 2 days.

Postoperative Treatment

We do NOT recommend administering nonsteroidal anti-inflammatory drugs to reduce pain after PTK because of their well-documented adverse effects on epithelial wound healing. After epithelial closure, topical antibiotics are typically not necessary any more. However, lubricants or gels and nonpreserved artificial tears should be applied to promote epithelial remodeling without long-lasting superficial punctate keratopathy. Typically topical steroids (e.g. fluorometholone 0.1% or prednisolone acetate 1% in the presence or likelihood of more profound stromal inflammation after deep ablation) are tapered slowly over some weeks or months. Depending on the depth of ablation, it might be started to be administered 4 times a day and reduced by 1 drop a day every month.

Indications and Outcome

In table 3, the potential indications for PTK are summarized. In the following paragraph, only some specific details and/or recommendations concerning PTK in certain corneal

Table 3. Indications for excimer laser PTK

Corneal dystrophies
Epithelial basement membrane dystrophy (synonyms: map-dot-fingerprint dystrophy)
Bowman's layer dystrophies
Reis-Bücklers corneal dystrophies
Thiel-Behnke corneal dystrophies
Meesmann-Wilke corneal dystrophies
Granular corneal dystrophies [1, 2]
Lattice corneal dystrophies
Macular corneal dystrophies
Schnyder corneal dystrophies
Recurrences on the graft after keratoplasty
(Bullous keratopathy in Fuchs corneal dystrophies; combination with amniotic membrane transplantation)
Other superficial corneal pathologies
Scars
Herpetic origin (never without systemic acyclovir!)
Adenoviral keratoconjunctivitis
Scrofulous
Following other corneal infections
Traumatic
Salzmann's nodular degeneration
Pterygium (with involvement of optical zone; without involvement of optical zone – no indication for PTK!)
Subepithelial band keratopathy
Mechanical scraping
EDTA chelating
PTK just for smoothing
Keratoconus
Fibroblastic subepithelial nodules ('proud nebulae')
Irregular astigmatism (but: biomechanical stability of the cornea may further be decreased) – in combination with riboflavin-UVA cross-linking
Persisting epithelial defects
Erosions
Ulcers
Recurrent corneal erosion syndrome
Trauma
Epithelial basal membrane dystrophy (synonyms: Cogan-Guerry variant)
Idiopathic

dystrophies are given. It must be stressed in advance that not the class of dystrophy itself but the individual distribution of opacification, the amount of surface irregularities and the degree of RCES in combination with subjective symptoms are determining the decision for or against and the individual modality of PTK in a given patient.

Criteria of Outcome

Morphology

At the conclusion of the PTK treatment the cornea typically has a ground-glass appearance. After epithelial healing, which is typically completed after 3–4 days, corneal luster is regained and visual acuity may be markedly increased despite residual opacities in the deep stroma.

Persisting focal opacifications (typically in the deeper stroma and in the corneal periphery) must be distinguished from 'haze' early after laser ablation and from recurrences of the dystrophy, which typically appear in the subepithelial area after some years depending on the type of dystrophy.

Function

Criteria to determine visual function after PTK include: (1) UCVA; (2) BCVA; (3) subjective refraction and spherical equivalent of refraction; (4) astigmatism (refractive cylinder and keratometric/topographic astigmatism); (5) central corneal power (keratometric/topographic); (6) contrast sensitivity, and (7) patient's subjective assessment (photophobia, halo, glare, ocular surface discomfort).

The goal of PTK is to improve BCVA by 2–5 lines. BCVA of 1.0 (20/20) is not the goal! In previously emmetropic or even hyperopic eyes, UCVA may be worse after PTK due to a hyperopic shift. Typically, topographic regularity of the corneal surface will be improved after PTK. 'Plus diseases' with prominent lesions are good candidates. In contrast, 'minus diseases' (localized depressed lesions, e.g. foreign body scars) are bad candidates.

Although one of the important goals of PTK is to obviate the need for PKP, corneal transplantation may still be necessary in some cases. We found that preceding PTK does not appear to impair the outcome of subsequent PKP in patients with macular and granular dystrophy [22].

Recurrent Erosions

To assess the effects of the e-PTK component (i.e. PTK to improve epithelial adhesion), the patient's subjective report on ocular surface discomfort is valuable. Other important outcome measures are time period until complete epithelial closure after PTK and recurrence rate of corneal erosions. This should not only be given as a percentage but also as Kaplan-Meier curves [8, 17].

Until now it is still unclear what the exact mechanism is by which interaction between UV light and corneal tissue during PTK results in better epithelial adherence. However, we were able to show that after PTK the number of hemidesmosomes is significantly increased (fig. 4) [25].

Meesmann Corneal Dystrophy

Meesmann corneal dystrophy is a rare bilateral autosomal dominant exclusively epithelial dystrophy that usually appears very early in life. Tiny epithelial vesicles can be seen

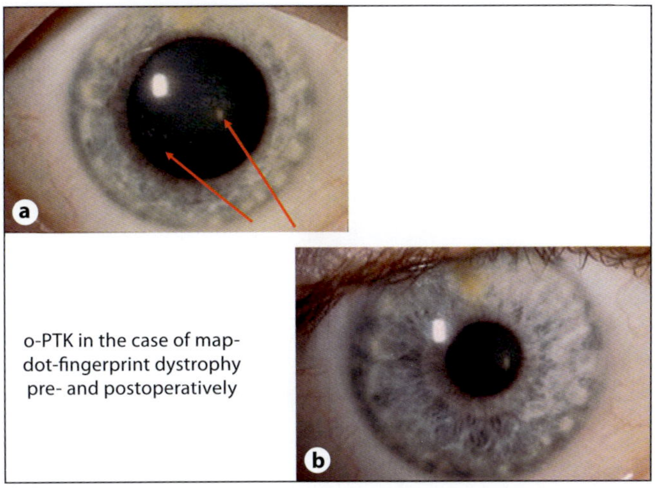

Fig. 5. Map-dot-fingerprint (epithelial basal membrane) corneal dystrophy: slit lamp appearance before excimer laser PTK (**a**), and no recurrence 4 years after excimer laser PTK (**b**) [8]. o-PTK = PTK to treat corneal opacity.

extending out to the limbus and may cause visual disturbance. Most patients are asymptomatic and hence require no treatment. Soft contact lens wear may help if patients show signs of RCES. Pure abrasion with a hockey knife should remove all the pathologic epithelium. Nevertheless, PTK may be used to enhance the adhesion of the corneal epithelium but results vary from good to bad with the possibility of inducing major haze [27].

Epithelial Basement Membrane Dystrophy

EBMD is the most common anterior corneal dystrophy [8, 20]. The so-called Cogan's microcystic dystrophy and the so-called map-dot-fingerprint dystrophy (Guerry) are variants or eponyms of EBMD. For both variants of EBMD, PTK using an excimer laser with low pulse energy and low number of pulses can be considered an effective and minimal invasive treatment modality to achieve a fast and durable epithelial closure, to prevent recurrent corneal erosions and to increase visual acuity in most patients (fig. 5) [8]. In this study, no recurrence of corneal erosion was observed during a mean follow-up of 4.8 years. Asymptomatic dystrophy signs in the midperiphery became visible in 2 out of 15 eyes at 3 and 5 years after PTK.

Granular Corneal Dystrophy

According to genetic studies, granular corneal dystrophy (GCD) is an epithelial rather than a stromal dystrophy. The multifocal opacities are usually superficial but can sometimes be located deeper in the stroma. In our department, GCD – besides RCES – was the dystrophy most frequently treated with PTK. To prevent a major hyperopic shift and to allow for repeat PTK in case of recurrence the primary ablation should be limited to less than 100 μm. The results are generally described as good (fig. 6) [9, 10].

Histomorphometric analysis of deposits in the cornea suggests that GCD is a better candidate than lattice dystrophy for PTK since the deposits are located more

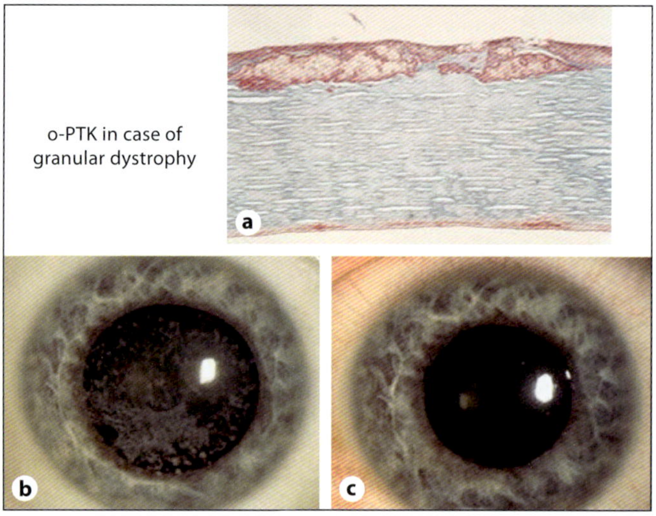

Fig. 6. GCD: superficial deposits of hyaline material (Masson's trichrome stain) (**a**), slit lamp appearance before excimer laser PTK (**b**), and 3 months after excimer laser PTK (**c**) [9]. o-PTK = PTK to treat corneal opacity.

superficially and the central clear optical zone after removal of 100 μm of tissue is significantly larger in granular (from 484 ± 389 μm to 1,451 ± 1,954 μm) than in lattice (from 258 ± 183 μm to 846 ± 784 μm) dystrophy. Deposits were completely removed in 22% of the GCD samples. In both dystrophies, a clear central 'pinhole' greater than 1 mm in diameter was achieved in around one third of corneas [3].

Lattice Corneal Dystrophy

Lattice corneal dystrophy (LCD) is characterized by the formation of branching filaments or bands in the corneal stroma. These are usually seen in the superficial part of the stroma, but it is not rare for them to penetrate deeper. The very center of the cornea is often opacified late in the disease but it is eventually overtaken by a general superficial opacification that reduces vision. Ablation of the superficial stroma removes the diffuse central opacity as well as some of the stromal branching filaments. Nevertheless, the average outcome in terms of visual acuity is decent but not impressive [9, 20]. The opacifications of LCD are often located too deeply to be completely removed. Spontaneous erosions are usual in LCD, but healing time is often longer than for other spontaneous erosions. In accordance, epithelial healing after PTK is typically delayed, too. It may require up to 3 weeks [28]. Recurrence rates are steady but fairly slow.

Bowman's Layer Dystrophies

Both types of Bowman's layer dystrophies have been confused for a long time. Both types are good candidates for PTK allowing for increased visual acuity and reduction of RCES. Eyes with Reis-Bücklers dystrophy seem to recur earlier than those with Thiel-Behnke dystrophy [20, 21].

Reis-Bücklers Corneal Dystrophy

RBCD is an autosomal dominant dystrophy where Bowman's layer is replaced with fibrocellular scar tissue that is classically described as 'saw tooth configuration'. The opacifications resemble geographic maps, but deposits reach deeper than in EBMD. PTK for RBCD is generally reported successful, but most recurrences appear within 1 year after PTK.

Thiel-Behnke Corneal Dystrophy

Thiel-Behnke corneal dystrophy (autosomal dominant inheritance) typically shows honeycomb opacifications of the superficial central stroma. In contrast to RBCD ('rod-shaped bodies'), Thiel-Behnke corneal dystrophy displays 'curly fibers' in Bowman's layer on transmission electron microscopic evaluation. Significant visual improvement may be achieved with PTK. Recurrences seem to appear more rarely and later than with RBCD.

Schnyder Corneal Dystrophy

Two changes characterize this dystrophy. One is a diffuse general, but not very dense opacification in the center of the corneal stroma. The other characteristic concerns the formation of subepithelial crystals in the center of the cornea in about half of the patients which scatter light very effectively. Schnyder corneal dystrophy is not very common. The treatment aims at removing the central superficial crystals. It seems that general stromal cloudiness does reduce vision to some extent as postoperative BCVA usually is about 20/40. However, visual acuity after PTK is maintained for a long time and recurrences seem to be very slow [20, 21, 27].

Macular Corneal Dystrophy

In the presence of superficial plaque-like opacities caused by macular corneal dystrophy PTK can moderately increase BCVA initially, although the diffusely scattered deep stromal opacities cannot be removed (fig. 7) [4]. In all patients with a follow-up of more than 1.4 years, a recurrence was observed leading to PKP in 6 of 10 eyes of this study. PTK should be considered after detailed explanation of limited long-term prognosis with the typically young patients (end of second decade). In addition, RCES may also be treated successfully by PTK. Despite possible complications primary PKP still seems to be the definite therapeutic option in patients with macular corneal dystrophy, because of the high recurrence rate after PTK and involvement of the corneal endothelium.

Recurrences of Dystrophies on Grafts after Keratoplasty

Various dystrophies seem to recur after different time periods following keratoplasty. Whereas GCD recurs very often and early, macular corneal dystrophy does recur very rarely and often not before 10–15 years after PKP.

In corneal grafts, the recurrence of GCD and LCD changes often take the form of superficial diffuse opacification (fig. 8). This type of opacification can be readily

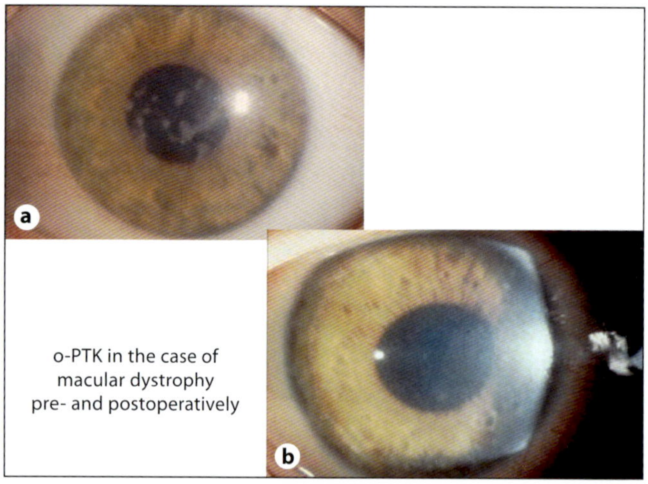

Fig. 7. Macular corneal dystrophy: slit lamp appearance before excimer laser PTK (**a**), and 6 weeks after excimer laser PTK (**b**). Note: only the superficial plaque-like opacifications can be removed with PTK [4]. o-PTK = PTK to treat corneal opacity.

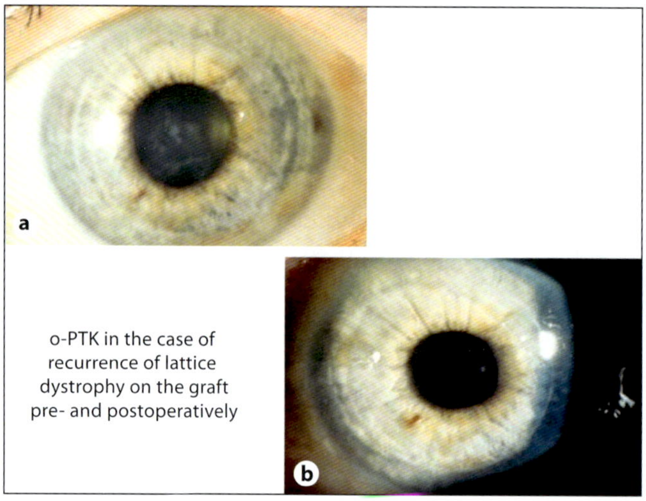

Fig. 8. Recurrence of LCD on the graft: slit lamp appearance before excimer laser PTK (**a**), and 6 months after excimer laser PTK (**b**). Be prepared for epithelial healing problems [28]. o-PTK = PTK to treat corneal opacity.

ablated and allow very acceptable vision for a few years. However, delayed epithelial healing has to be taken into account in LCD [28].

On a corneal graft, simultaneous correction of high astigmatism (in part) may be considered [29, 30]. In addition, prophylactic systemic corticosteroids may be helpful to avoid the induction of an immunologic graft rejection due to PTK [31, 32].

Fuchs Endothelial Corneal Dystrophy

Fuchs endothelial corneal dystrophy (FECD) is by definition an inherited disease. With progressive endothelial dysfunction due to increasing cornea guttata, it results in bullous keratopathy. There is no doubt that either PKP or posterior lamellar

Table 4. Complications of excimer laser PTK

Delayed epithelial healing (especially in lattice dystrophy)
Refractive and topographic changes
Hyperopic sift
Paradoxical myopic shift
Irregular astigmatism
Decentration
Stromal haze and scarring
Infectious ulcer/melting/perforation
Immunologic allograft rejection after PKP
Recurrence of disease
Corneal ectasia
Reactivation of herpes simplex keratitis
Intraocular lens power calculation for cataract surgery in eyes after PTK
(Subsequent penetrating keratoplasty needed)

keratoplasty are the treatment options of choice in eyes with good visual prognosis. However, in cases of low visual prognosis or patients with major noncompliance, superficial excimer laser ablation may be a palliative option. One of the rationales for PTK in bullous keratopathy is the chance to improve vision by ablating subepithelial scar tissue. However, exaggerated wound healing may lead to increased corneal scarring in those eyes [33]. Another reason for PTK concerns alleviation of pain. For this purpose, deeper ablation of up to 100 μm seems to be more effective than a more superficial approach. A combination with amniotic membrane transplantation (graft technique to ensure integration of amniotic membrane into the cornea) may even improve the outcome. Postoperatively, a long-term therapeutic contact lens seems to be helpful.

Complications

Three postoperative healing stages may be distinguished following PTK: (1) reepithelialization takes from 3–4 days (normal) to a few weeks (delayed) in some patients; (2) stromal remodeling occurs over the succeeding weeks and months, and (3) stabilization of topography and refractive changes may take months. Consequently, general postoperative goals include encouragement of epithelialization, minimization of stromal scarring and optimization of refractive and topographic outcome. Potential complications after PTK [34] are listed in table 4.

Delayed Epithelial Healing

Patients who have suffered previous ocular surface disease with loss of epithelial vitality may have problems with epithelialization following PTK. Eyes with severe ocular surface diseases such as chemical burns, ocular cicatricial pemphigoid, atopic kerato-conjunctivitis and severe dysfunctional tear syndrome should be treated with extreme caution – if at all. However, even in eyes with 'pure corneal dystrophy' delayed epithelial healing may occur.

We performed a study to evaluate the time period necessary for complete epithelial healing after PTK carried out for various superficial corneal opacities [28]. One hundred and ninety-seven eyes were divided into 9 groups. One hundred and sixty-one eyes (95%) healed within 7 days. Overall, 63, 80, and 85% of epithelial defects were closed within 3, 4 and 5 days, respectively. Out of 9 eyes which showed delayed healing, 6 eyes (67%) belonged to the LCD category. The mean time taken for healing in the LCD group (8.6 ± 8.4 days) was significantly longer than in all other groups (mean 2.7±3.7 days). Besides adequate counseling, these patients with LCD should be followed up closely until complete closure of the epithelium to avoid ulceration, scarring or even infection.

In general, potential reasons for delayed epithelial healing include: (1) systemic rheumatoid diseases (e.g. lupus erythematosus); (2) toxicity of topical medication (e.g. nonsteroidal anti-inflammatory drugs, steroids, gentamycin, preservatives); (3) presence of preoperative active ocular surface and lid inflammatory disease; (4) dry eye or dysfunctional tear syndrome, and (5) denervation after PKP. Those eyes with LCD might need additional treatment (perhaps prophylactic) such as hyaluronic acid drops, autologous blood serum drops [14], a bandage soft contact lens, punctal plugs/occlusion, simultaneous amniotic membrane patching or even temporary lateral tarsorrhaphy or botulinum toxin injection to induce a temporary ptosis. Lid surgery to correct malposition should preferably be performed before PTK.

Refractive and Topographic Changes

Ablation of the corneal surface will lead to refractive and topographic changes after PTK. Such effects may be predicted by the type of corneal disorder treated and the surgical strategy employed. The anticipated refractive changes should be considered during surgical decision making and strategic planning of technical details. Today, simultaneous hyperopic/astigmatic or even topography-based refractive ablation may be performed with acceptable results.

Hyperopic Shift

When performing PTK – at least with a broad-beam laser – the laser beam is of a fixed diameter. Since the energy is optimally homogeneous over the face, the ablation rate would theoretically be similar over the treated area of the cornea. Thus, with a direct ablation without polishing, the surface profile would be expected to be preserved without change in corneal power or topography, and the refraction similarly would be expected to be unchanged. However, studies and clinical practice indicate that a hyperopic shift is a frequent concomitant of PTK procedures [35]. There are several hypotheses to explain this phenomenon as outlined below.

1 The full-spot (= wide-field) laser beam in practice may exhibit somewhat attenuated fluence ('beam inhomogeneity') at its peripheral aspect. Thus, the peripheral ablation rate may be slightly less militating towards corneal flattening.
2 The induced corneal flattening may be caused by an unequal postoperative epithelial thickness with creation of an epithelial lens power different from the curvature of the underlying treated stroma. Epithelial hyperplasia at the periphery of the treated area could be implicated as a cause, especially if a metal mask is used to protect peripheral Bowman's layer.
3 The changing angle of incidence of the beam across the corneal dome might result in a lower fluence peripherally with a decrease in effective tissue ablation and consequent corneal flattening. An analogous phenomenon may result when focusing the laser on the apex of the cornea with the consequence of a peripheral defocus with potentially less tissue ablation. Both aspects may be of questionable clinical impact.
4 Other researchers suggest that removal of the central portion of corneal stroma lamellae may lead to centrifugal differential contraction of the remaining peripheral superficial lamellae with consequent central flattening. Dupps and Roberts [36] favor the model of differential swelling of midperipheral collagen fibers after removal of central superficial stromal tissue.
5 In addition, a peripheral meniscus of masking fluid (especially when using a metal mask) may prevent the (mid-)peripheral corneal tissue from being ablated to the same extent as the central tissue.
6 It may also be speculated that the laser plume may differentially block the periphery of the incoming beam thus leading to less peripheral ablation.

Paradoxical Myopic Shift

Steepening of the central cornea may occur when more tissue is removed peripherally than centrally. Although this may flatten the focal area of the cornea treated due to mechanisms discussed above, the overall optical contour of the cornea may steepen if peripheral tissue is removed. Typically, a paradoxical myopic shift occurs after removal of peripheral prominent pannus with the hockey knife before laser action (e.g. in case of Salzmann's nodular degeneration).

Irregular Astigmatism (Focal Ablation)

PTK to improve the adherence of the epithelium is supposed to smoothen the surface and reduce preexisting irregular astigmatism. However, irregular astigmatism may be induced inadvertently during the laser procedure. This may be caused by decentration of the ablation, which should be centered on the entrance pupil – not on the center of the pathology. If the pathology covers only half of the pupil, it is indispensable to ablate undiseased tissue to avoid irregular astigmatism. Uneven distribution of masking fluid with inadequately high viscosity may also result in focal hyperablation and irregular astigmatism. Typically, epithelial remodeling is able to compensate for some degree of irregular astigmatism by focal hyperplasia and focal hypoplasia. However, this helpful mechanism may take some months.

Haze/Scars

In general, PTK has as one of its primary goals the amelioration of corneal opacity. Thus, postoperative stromal haze is of less concern for PTK than for PRK. Efforts promoting prompt closure of the epithelium should mitigate an adverse stromal wound healing response. In addition, adjunctive use of topical corticosteroids may also be helpful in avoiding excessive keratocyte activation and scar formation.

Early after PTK, a trace to mild reticular subepithelial stromal haze seems to be quite common. The intensity seems to depend on the depth of ablation and it seems to fade away over a few months. In case of preexisting scars, the probability of renewed scar formation is higher. In these eyes, the application of mitomycin C should be considered [26].

Infectious Ulcer/Melting/Perforation

The risk of microbial keratitis due to the iatrogenic introduction of an epithelial defect is very low, but this is a serious complication that can quite adversely affect the final visual outcome [37]. The greatest risk of microbial keratitis following PTK is either before reepithelialization is complete or within the first few weeks after reepithelialization before the risk of recurrent erosion is virtually eliminated. Moreover, the previously diseased cornea is at greater risk of infection following surgery than the healthy cornea. Persisting epithelial defects in such eyes may afford an inviting substrate for microbial keratitis. Thus, infection will be discouraged with prompt reepithelialization of the defect and strenuous efforts should be made to avoid persisting epithelial defects. We apply nonpreserved fluoroquinolone antibiotics as a routine after PTK because they are much less toxic to the epithelium than aminoglycosides. Following PTK, the patient should be closely followed in the face of a persistent epithelial defect especially if a bandage soft contact lens is in place. Any infiltrate and infection should promptly be treated with broad-spectrum antibiotic coverage or so-called 'fortified drops'.

In analogy to refractive surgery, systemic vasculitis or collagenolytic disease (e.g. Morbus Wegener, rheumatoid arthritis, systemic lupus erythematodes) are contraindications, because the cornea may melt resulting in a (perforated) nonreactive ulcer.

Immunologic Allograft Rejection after Penetrating Keratoplasty

Immunologic graft rejection after PKP may be prompted by any surgical procedure on the graft. PTK may be such a procedure, especially in case of provoked inflammation due to a prolonged time period until epithelial closure. There have been cases of immunologic graft rejection after PTK reported in the literature [31, 32]. It may happen even years after PKP. Although it is unclear what precipitated the immune reaction (laser treatment itself, manual epithelial removal, alterations in the patient's medical regimen), it is clear, however, that immediate topical and systemic treatment with corticosteroids is indispensable to manage this rare complication after PTK. It should be considered to administer a moderate dose of systemic corticosteroid (e.g. 80 mg prednisolone acetate orally) for a few days after PTK on a corneal graft as a prophylaxis.

Recurrence of Disease

Patients with corneal dystrophies undergoing PTK may suffer recurrences following the procedure. Disorders such as lattice/granular/macular corneal dystrophy, EBMD or Salzmann's nodular degeneration may recur at variable intervals after PTK. It is important to inform the patient of this possibility. PTK or manual superficial keratectomy while clearing and smoothing the cornea does not cure the underlying disorder of the epithelium or keratocytes. In cases where the disease presents itself again and becomes visually significant, PTK can be repeated as long as enough corneal tissue is available.

Our clinical impression based on scientific evaluation is that recurrences on the original cornea after PTK behave differently when compared to recurrences of the same dystrophy on the graft after transplantation: while granular dystrophy recurs quite often and quickly on the graft [6], it recurs late after PTK [9]. While macular dystrophy recurs after decades on the graft, superficial plaque-like opacities recur very quickly after PTK [4]. In contrast, map-dot-fingerprint dystrophy recurs very late. Some eyes did not show a morphologic recurrence of RCES after 9 years [8]. Presenting studies on recurrences of dystrophies after PTK should include cumulative Kaplan-Meier recurrence rates, not only relative risk as a percentage.

Reactivation of herpetic/adenoviral disease may be induced by UV light effects during PTK [38, 39]. Besides laser effects, manual trauma and postoperative use of corticosteroids may be factors in herpes reactivation. This may be true in case of concomitant corneal scars after herpetic keratitis. Thus, active herpes keratitis is an absolute, herpetic scars a relative contraindication for PTK. If PTK is performed on a herpetic scar, a quiescent period of 6–12 months is preferred before PTK and perioperative treatment with topical antiviral agents as well as oral acyclovir may act as prophylaxis against recurrent herpetic infection.

Corneal Ectasia

Corneas that are too thin (i.e. <400 μm) should not be treated with the laser, since additional tissue removal may destabilize the corneal biomechanics or may further distort the corneal surface with the consequence of progressive myopia. In addition, deep laser ablation may damage corneal endothelium by concomitant shock waves. An analogous problem may appear after PRK or laser-assisted in situ keratomileusis (LASIK) with too thin a residual stromal bed thickness [40].

Intraocular Lens Power Calculation for Cataract Surgery after Phototherapeutic Keratectomy

For more than one decade, it has been well known that intraocular lens power calculation after myopic PRK/LASIK results in postoperative hyperopia if no precautions are taken. The deviation from the intended spherical equivalent increases with the amount of the myopic correction that precedes [41]. Since PTK inadvertently results in flattening of the cornea, this problem may also apply here – to some extent. Cataract surgeons should know about this potential risk of intraocular lens miscalculation after PTK. Nevertheless, patients after PTK are typically much less demanding than patients after PRK/LASIK in terms of achieving an optimal UCVA after phakoemulsification.

Anterior Lamellar Keratoplasty

Introduction

In case of deeper corneal stromal deposits sparing the endothelium, such as in special variants of granular or lattice dystrophy, PTK may not be sufficient whereas PKP may appear to be 'overtreatment'. In these cases, ALKP can be considered [42].

ALKP was developed more than 150 years ago [43, 44]. The first attempt to dissect near Descemet's membrane, in the sense of deep anterior lamellar keratoplasty (DALK), was described by Hallermann [44]. The main disadvantage of DALK is that it is both a technically more challenging and time-consuming procedure with a steep learning curve compared with PKP with a high possibility of Descemet's membrane perforations, particularly when the host stroma is manually removed layer by layer until the Descemet's membrane is exposed [45]. Another reason for surgeons to perform a PKP for anterior corneal disorders is that lamellar transplants often show decreased BCVA owing to irregular astigmatism and/or scarring at the donor-to-recipient interface [46, 47].

Archila [48] and Anwar [49] were the first to describe complete baring of Descemet's membrane in the recipient cornea. This technique promised to result in less interface opacity and hence improved visual acuity postoperatively, yielding vision comparable to that resulting from PKP. As concluded by Anwar [50] in 1972 when he described the dissection technique for ALKP, lamellar transplants are more advantageous since they are followed by fewer complications as the globe is not opened. Also, the donor material does not have to be as fresh as that required in full-thickness keratoplasty. He stressed the importance of improving the visual results of the lamellar operation as well as making it the first-choice intervention if the endothelium is found to be healthy.

Technique of Deep Anterior Lamellar Keratoplasty

Some corneal surgeons suggest starting by performing a separate corneal incision, 1 mm inside the limbus, using a 550-μm guarded limbal relaxing incision knife or

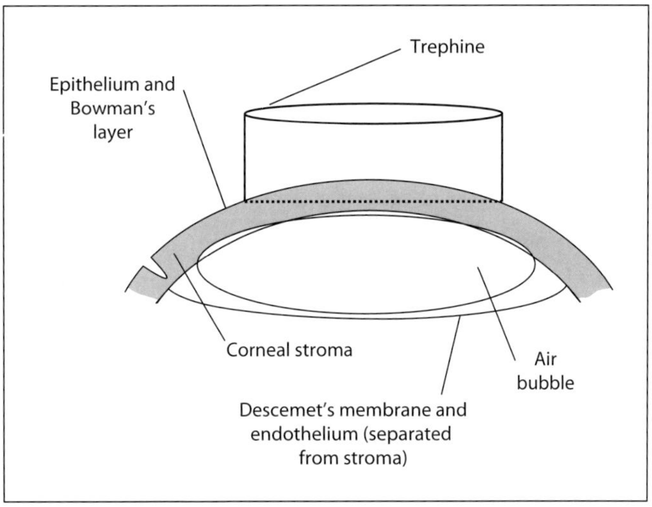

Fig. 9. Trephination of the recipient stroma after creating the air bubble separating Descemet's membrane in DALK.

even the femtosecond laser after performing pachymetry. A peripheral paracentesis is performed. Then a 27- or 30-gauge needle is attached to a 1- to 3-ml air-filled syringe. The needle is bent approximately 5.0 mm from its tip so that the terminal segment angles up approximately 60° while the bevel faces down. The tip is introduced, bevel down, into the corneal stroma at the chosen entry site, in the depth of the incision. Under direct visual control, the needle is carefully advanced towards the center of the cornea in a direction halfway between a tangential and a radial one until the bevel is completely buried, about 3.0 mm from the entry point. Air is injected progressively into the stroma, with the aim of achieving the formation of a large air bubble between the Descemet's membrane and stroma extending as peripheral as possible (fig. 9). This usually appears in the form of a white disk starting near the tip of the needle and gradually enlarging towards the periphery of the cornea. If no bubble is formed, air injection can be repeated by reentering from the incision site. When a sufficiently large bubble is achieved, a small amount of aqueous is allowed to escape to lower the intraocular pressure.

The size of trephination of the recipient bed is determined aiming to surround the entire superficial stromal pathology. Partial-thickness trephination of the cornea is performed to a depth between 350 and 400 μm using a Hanna suction trephine (Moria, France), the Guided Trephine System (GTS, Polytech, Germany) or a Hessburg-Barron vacuum trephine, which is less precise [12] but easy to use and disposable [51–53]. Lamellar superficial keratectomy is performed with a crescent knife aiming to leave a layer of corneal stroma in place anterior to the air bubble. A 15° slit knife is inserted into the large bubble, allowing the air to escape and collapsing the bubble. Viscoelastic material is injected from the opening done by the knife. Then the stroma is removed by blunt-tipped scissors.

The donor cornea is punched out from the endothelial side with a Hanna donor punch or a Barron donor punch (0.25 mm oversize) or from the epithelial side using the GTS (same size). The Descemet's membrane with endothelium is gently stripped off with a dry Weck-Cel sponge or using a forceps. The button is sutured in place using a double-running cross-stitch suture according to Hoffmann after copiously irrigating the Descemet's membrane to wash away all viscoelastic material.

Postoperative medications included topical prednisolone acetate 1% 4 times daily for 1 month, gradually tapered over 6 months, ofloxacin eyedrops 4 times daily for 1 week, and artificial tear preparations 4–6 times daily.

Discussion

DALK is a relatively new technique of lamellar corneal transplantation surgery used to treat corneal diseases that do not involve Descemet's membrane [54]. The technique allows the placement of a nearly full-thickness corneal donor button onto the host bed containing minimal or no stromal tissue on Descemet's membrane and is preferred over performing PKP for treating corneal stromal pathologies. It avoids the replacement of host endothelium with donor endothelium, thus removing the main antigenic load reducing the incidence of graft rejection. Also, it has less effect on endothelial cell count [55].

Other advantages of DALK over PKP as a treatment for corneal stromal disease are those of a lamellar procedure: avoiding most complications associated with 'open-sky' surgery, less chances of intraoperative complications such as expulsive hemorrhage and postoperative complications such as anterior synechiae or secondary glaucoma. Thus, DALK retains all the advantages of lamellar keratoplasty over PKP while providing a clear interface compared with that of conventional 'midstromal' lamellar keratoplasty.

In an attempt to facilitate dissection, Melles et al. [56] in 1999 injected air into the anterior chamber to improve visualization of Descemet's membrane during dissection. They started the dissection through a scleral incision 1 mm outside the limbus, and injected viscoelastic material in the dissected pocket before trephination. A more recent study by Marchini et al. [57] in 2006 used a similar technique, but started dissection from a limbal incision, using a specially designed set of instruments.

Although better microkeratomes have become available with the development of LASIK, microkeratome lamellar resections cannot be used for disorders with deep stromal opacities, variable corneal thickness, and surface irregularities [58]. The use of the femtosecond laser in fashioning the donor and recipient corneal lenticules faces the same problem of equipment availability (laser machine and artificial anterior chamber or whole donor globe) in addition to the expenses [59].

The technique of injecting air into the corneal stroma to facilitate dissection down to the Descemet's membrane led to reduced interface haze and better postoperative visual results. However, the rate of intraoperative perforation was high (39.2%) [57]. Descemet's membrane separation is essential in improving the postoperative visual function, as stated by Ardjomand et al. [60]. They suggested that the main parameter for good visual function after DALK for keratoconus is the thickness of the residual recipient stromal bed. DALK performed in an eye with a residual bed thickness of <20 μm can achieve a similar visual result as PKP, whereas the eyes with a recipient stromal bed thickness of >80 μm had a significantly reduced visual acuity.

In contrast to the other described techniques of ALKP, the big-bubble technique creates a perfect cleavage plane between Descemet's membrane and the rest of the corneal tissue and appears to be much safer than the manual technique of achieving deep stromal dissection regarding the incidence of macroperforations. The big-bubble technique also ensures a maximum possible depth dissection achieving a complete baring of Descemet's membrane so that no stromal tissue is left to cause interface haze in the future [61].

The importance of maintaining an intact Descemet's membrane was proven by Den et al. [62]. They found that the rate of endothelial decompensation was higher in patients with Descemet's membrane perforation. They attributed this to either direct insult to the cells associated with perforation or the ensuing pseudochamber formation or gas tamponade.

In case Descemet's membrane separation is not achieved or in case of macroperforation, the procedure is converted to a full-thickness transplantation. Using the excimer laser for lamellar trephination along metal masks, conversion to PKP can be performed without any disadvantage to the patient [63].

Posterior Lamellar Keratoplasty

Introduction

In case of solitary endothelial dystrophies, such as FECD, posterior polymorphous corneal dystrophy or even congenital hereditary endothelial dystrophy, only the diseased parts of the cornea may be replaced.

Today the procedure most widely applied is Descemet stripping automated endothelial keratoplasty (DSAEK). This technique refers to only removing Descemet's membrane in the recipient and then adding the transplant consisting of a thin stromal layer, Descemet's membrane and endothelium. 'Automated' refers to those techniques employing a microkeratome for preparation of the donor lamella [64–66].

In some centers, Descemet membrane endothelial keratoplasty (DMEK) is being tested, which includes removing the Descemet's membrane in the recipient and transplanting the Descemet's membrane and endothelium only [67]. This technique, still being under development, is obviously the most desirable from a theoretical standpoint, but needs further refinement before it can be introduced into routine clinical application due to major endothelial cell loss and technical difficulties potentially resulting in a major waste of precious donor tissue.

Advantages and Disadvantages of Posterior Lamellar Keratoplasty

The main advantages of posterior lamellar keratoplasty are [68]:

1 mechanical stability of cornea/globe basically unaltered;
2 fast visual rehabilitation;
3 almost neutral procedure concerning refraction;
4 'sutureless' procedure and therefore no suture-related complications;
5 intact corneal innervation;
6 lower risk of late wound dehiscence;
7 surgical procedure through small incisions in a closed system and thus less theoretical risk of choroidal hemorrhage and infection;
8 transplantation of less allogenic material and therefore less theoretical risk of graft rejection;
9 possibility of PKP remains if lamellar procedure does not satisfy the patient's visual needs;
10 repeatability of the transplantation.

The main disadvantages are (1) the problem inherent to all lamellar techniques, which is the construction of an interface with its negative impact on final visual acuity, and (2) the high amount of endothelial cell loss with current surgical techniques, which is attributed to the need for excessive manipulation of donor endothelium [65, 68].

Technique of Descemet Stripping Automated Endothelial Keratoplasty

First, an endothelial transplant is created by cutting a deep 'free' flap over the center of a donor cornea on an artificial anterior chamber and then punching the desired size (e.g. 9 mm) of the transplant from the endothelial side. After creating two opposite clear corneal incisions in the recipient, the Descemet's membrane is scored circularly and subsequently removed in the central corneal area with a special spatula ('stripping'). Then the transplant is introduced into the anterior chamber with various techniques, which all involve some kind of folding of the lamella. The transplant is then pressed against the back of the corneal stroma by injecting an air bubble into the anterior chamber, which may be partly removed at the end of surgery. The patient may then be advised to remain in back position (in order to press the transplant against the corneal back surface by the air bubble) depending on the surgeon. It may be advisable for the patient to lay down on his/her back until the next morning and have an Nd:YAG iridotomy performed preoperatively or a surgical iridotomy/

iridectomy intraoperatively to prevent papillary block with the consequence of dramatic pressure rise.

Indication and Limitations for Descemet Stripping Automated Endothelial Keratoplasty in Fuchs Endothelial Corneal Dystrophy

The principal requirement for successful posterior lamellar grafting is that the corneal stroma and surface be free of alterations which significantly impair vision (e.g. opacities or irregularities).

In partly or completely decompensated corneas, vision will usually be severely impaired and many patients will be symptomatic with edematous epithelium and with rupture of epithelial bullae. In these cases, the loose epithelium should be removed intraoperatively but the indication for surgery is usually straightforward.

In corneas in which guttae are present without decompensation, but to a degree/density which is visually symptomatic – especially by deterioration of contrast sensitivity – indication for surgery is relative and dependent on individual visual needs and demands of the patient.

Performing either penetrating or lamellar surgery is currently a matter of evolving opinion formation.

(1) In eyes with pronounced bullous keratopathy and symptomatology from discomfort to pain, DSAEK may be preferable – at least as a first-line treatment. If such eyes have reduced visual potential for other reasons than the corneal decompensation, the palliative indication being more or less prominent in the decision-making process, the lamellar option may also be superior. Even if the visual potential is full or close to it, lamellar surgery will have priority in older patients and those with average visual demand, while the potential for optimal and long-term visual result and endothelial survival is to be considered mainly in young and visually demanding patients.

(2) In patients/eyes with compensated corneal guttata, the above considerations require even more individual weighing of the above factors.

(3) In case of corneal opacities or irregularities, which would impede vision despite elimination of corneal edema, the penetrating option should be considered in accordance with the criteria outlined above [69].

Postoperative Course, Care and Complications

Once the transplant stays attached in the anterior chamber without air tamponade, it will not detach. Postoperative clarity of the recipient cornea usually occurs within days, resulting in 'useful' vision quickly. Over the following weeks, vision will gradually improve further. With full functional potential, vision may increase to >20/40 in about 80% of cases within a few months – but being highly dependent on the

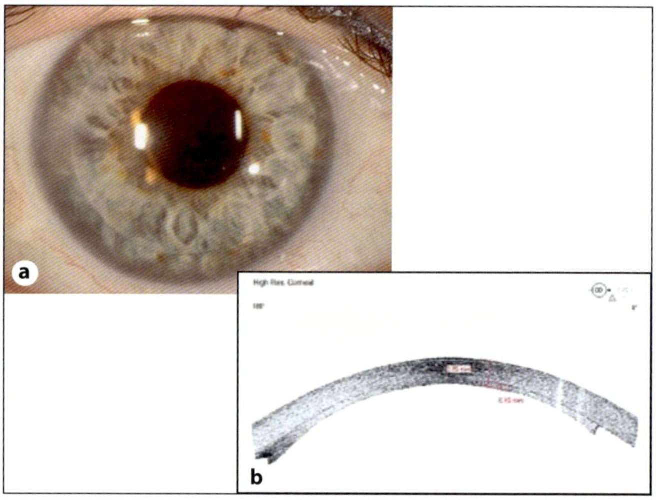

Fig. 10. DSAEK in FECD. **a** Anterior segment of an eye with an endothelial transplant. The transplant can bee seen as a round contour, attached to the inner corneal surface – without sutures. **b** Optical coherence pachymetry demonstrating a sagittal section through a cornea with an endothelial transplant (0.15 mm) after DSAEK [69].

surgeon's individual technique. Visual acuity of 20/25 may be achieved very rarely (fig. 10a) [70].

Postoperative treatment usually consists of topical steroids tapered over 6 months. Basically, the same criteria apply as after PKP. The rate of immune reactions seems to be in the same range as with PKP. Refractive changes introduced by the procedure usually consist of a slight hyperopic shift, which may be explained by the optical effect of the meniscus shape of the transplanted 'lenticule' (fig. 10b), i.e. it induced negative dioptric power [70, 71].

DSAEK can be combined with cataract surgery. In these cases, intraocular lens power calculation should account for the induced hyperopic shift (around 1.0–1.25 dpt). Nevertheless, the DSAEK procedure is preferably performed in primary pseudophakic eyes – especially during the learning curve of the microsurgeon.

To date there is no evidence for an artificially high intraocular pressure due to the thicker cornea after endothelial keratoplasty measured with Goldmann applanation tonometry [72].

Penetrating Keratoplasty

The classical option and gold standard in the surgical treatment of FECD has been PKP [73, 74]. Typically, our cutoff visual acuity for surgery is around 20/50 (0.4). However, we do modify this according to the needs of the patient. The outcome of PKP in FECD is generally good, due to the primary lack of vascularization, inflammation, uneven corneal thickness or other disadvantageous prognostic factors [75]. The 10-year graft survival in this condition has been reported as high as 80–90% in a recent series [76]. The risk profile of this intervention includes prolonged visual rehabilitation, high astigmatism, suture-related complications, wound dehiscence and immunologic graft rejection. To date the reason for an ongoing idiopathic endothelial cell loss which occurs in the graft is unclear [77].

Alternative Treatment Options in Fuchs Endothelial Corneal Dystrophy

Early stages of cornea guttata do not require any therapy at all. Patients should be counseled accordingly. Visually significant corneal edema is symptomatically treated with topical hyperosmotic agents such as 5% NaCl drops 4–6 times a day. Application is to be started in the morning upon awaking to promote early vision increase. In addition, artificial tears or gels during daytime and ointment at night might help to prevent bullous keratopathy from becoming painful. In case of bullous keratopathy, a bandage soft contact lens is typically helpful. In these cases, additional topical application of nonpreserved antibiotics (typically fluorochinolones) is advisable.

Several palliative options have been proposed for painful bullous keratopathy in case no corneal transplant is available. They include anterior stromal puncture, amniotic membrane transplantation as a graft – not only a patch [78]. This may or may not be combined with aggressive PTK to strengthen the adhesions between epithelium and superficial stroma.

Techniques of Penetrating Keratoplasty

A few general technical details concerning PKP need to be addressed [63, 73].

1. Donor topography should be attempted for exclusion of previous refractive surgery, keratoconus/high astigmatism.
2. General anesthesia has advantages over local anesthesia. The arterial blood pressure should be kept low as the eye is opened ('controlled arterial hypotension').
3. Donor and recipient trephination should be performed from the epithelial side with the same system, which is the predisposition for congruent cut surfaces and angles in donor and recipient. For this purpose, an artificial anterior chamber is used for donor trephination.
4. Graft size should be adjusted individually ('as large as possible, as small as necessary') [79].
5. Excessive graft over- or undersize should be avoided to prevent stretching or compression of peripheral donor tissue.
6. Horizontal positioning of head and limbal plane are indispensable for state-of-the-art PKP surgery in order to avoid decentration and vertical tilt.
7. Limbal centration should be preferred over pupil centration.

8 To protect the crystalline lens in phakic keratoplasty, usually the pupil is constricted.
9 Before recipient trephination, a paracentesis at the limbus is performed.
10 An optional iridotomy prevents pupillary block and acute angle closure glaucoma (so-called 'Urrets-Zavalia syndrome') in case of dilated pupil with iris sphincter necrosis.
11 The second cardinal suture exactly 180° away from the first suture is crucial for symmetrical graft alignment and to avoid horizontal torsion.
12 Orientation structures in the donor and host facilitate the correct placement of the first 8 cardinal sutures to avoid horizontal torsion.
13 As long as Bowman's layer is intact, a double-running cross-stitch suture (according to Hoffmann) is preferred since it results in higher topographic regularity, earlier visual rehabilitation and less suture loosening requiring only rarely additional suture replacement.
14 Intraoperative keratoscopy should be applied after removal of lid specula and fixation sutures. Unstable donor epithelium should better be removed to allow for reproducible results. Adjustment of double-running sutures or replacement of single sutures may be indicated.

Technique of Nonmechanical Excimer Laser Trephination for Penetrating Keratoplasty
A measurable improvement of PKP results seems to be possible, using the Krumeich GTS, the second-generation Hanna trephine and our technique of nonmechanical trephination with the excimer laser [80, 81]. Since 1989 more than 3,000 human eyes have been treated successfully with the Meditec MEL60® excimer laser in Homburg/Saar and Erlangen. Besides keratoconus, FECD has been by far the leading indication for PKP with this noncontact technique [82].

The main advantage of this novel laser cutting technique performed from the epithelial side in the donor and recipient is – in contrast to the femtosecond laser application – the avoidance of mechanical distortion by applanation during trephination, resulting in smooth cut edges which are congruent in the donor and patient potentially reducing 'vertical tilt'. Such cut edges in combination with 'orientation teeth' [83] at the graft margin and corresponding notches at the recipient margin for symmetric positioning of the 8 cardinal sutures minimizes 'horizontal torsion', thus potentially improving the optical performance after transplantation (fig. 11). Furthermore, recipient and donor decentration may be reduced [84]. The use of metal masks allows for arbitrary shapes of the trephination, e.g. elliptical [85].

These favorable impacts on major intraoperative determinants of postkeratoplasty astigmatism result in lower keratometric astigmatism, higher topographic regularity and better visual acuity after suture removal (table 5) [81, 86, 87]. After sequential removal of a double-running suture, keratometric astigmatism increased in 80% of eyes with conventional trephination, but further decreased in 52% of eyes with laser trephination.

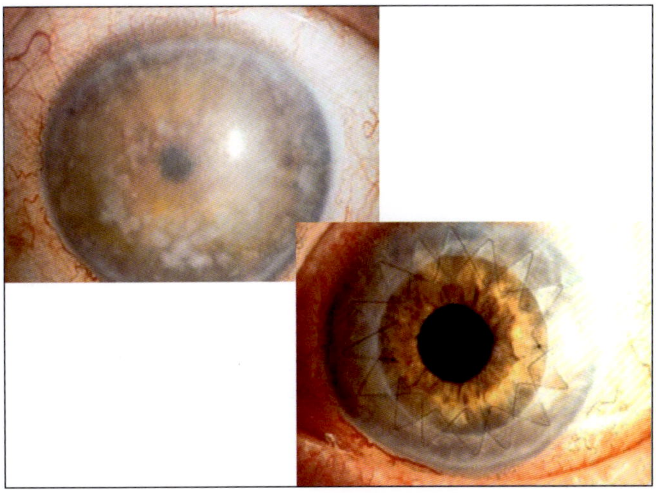

Fig. 11. Typical double-running 10-0 nylon cross-stitch suture with 8 bites each (according to Hoffmann) in macular dystrophy (7.5/7.6 mm, excimer laser trephination with 8 'orientation teeth/notches').

Table 5. Advantages of nonmechanical trephination with the 193-nm excimer laser along metal masks with 'orientation teeth/notches'

No trauma to intraocular tissues
Avoid deformation and compression of tissue during trephination
Reduction of horizontal torsion ('orientation teeth/notches')
Reduction of vertical tilt (congruent cut edges)
Reduction of host and donor decentration
Feasibility of 'harmonization' of donor and host topography
Reduction of anterior chamber inflammation early after PKP
Reduction of astigmatism after suture removal
Higher regularity of corneal topography
Significantly better visual acuity with spectacle correction
Feasibility of trephination with instable cornea (e.g. 'open eye', descemetocele, after radial keratotomy, iatrogenic keratectasia after LASIK)
Arbitrary shape (e.g. elliptical)

Options of Femtosecond Laser Trephination for Penetrating Keratoplasty

Recently, the options for PKP have been expanded to include femtosecond laser-assisted trephination of contoured wound configurations. With this option, the construction of the recipient and donor can be adjusted to the requirements of the disease. For FECD, the so-called 'inverse mushroom' [88] or 'top hat' [89, 90] configuration of the transplant has been proposed, which describes a shape with a larger diameter on the endothelial side and a smaller diameter on the epithelial side (fig. 12). The main advantage of the contoured/shaped grafts is that less 'unnecessary' (in this case epithelium and anterior stroma) tissue is transplanted, and that

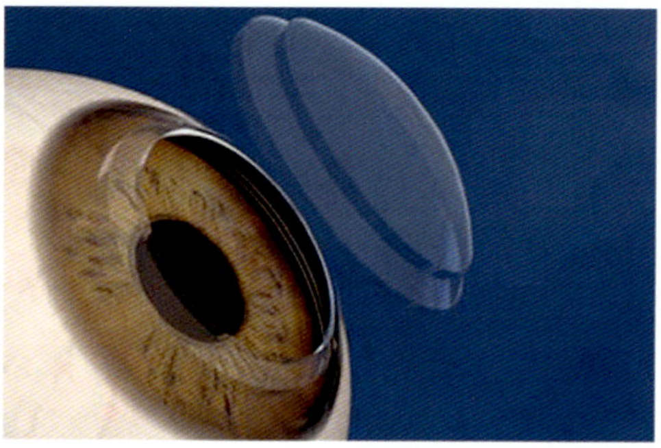

Fig. 12. Drawing of a 'top hat' = 'inverse mushroom' trephination using a femtosecond laser for PKP. The unsolved problem is the applanation of host cornea during trephination.

this wound configuration provides superior sealing characteristics thus being more stable against pressure [89, 90]. The major disadvantage of this technique is the need of suction and applanation of the cornea. At this time, no results concerning objective keratometric astigmatism with and without sutures, regularity of graft topography, and BCVA after suture removal are available in the literature in this exciting new field of corneal transplant surgery.

The Triple Procedure

Since the introduction of the triple procedure (= simultaneous PKP, extracapsular cataract extraction and implantation of a posterior chamber intraocular lens) in the mid-seventies, there has been an ongoing discussion among corneal microsurgeons concerning the best approach (simultaneous or sequential) for combined corneal disease and cataract [91, 92]. For the refractive results after the triple procedure, some intraoperative details are crucial: trephination of the recipient and donor from the epithelial side without major oversize (GTS or nonmechanical excimer laser trephination) should preserve the preoperative corneal curvature in FECD. The graft and the posterior chamber intraocular lens placed in the bag after large continuous curvilinear capsulorhexis should be centered along the optical axis. If possible, performing capsulorhexis under controlled intraocular pressure conditions prior to trephination may help to minimize the risk of capsular ruptures. In case of excessive corneal clouding, a capsulorhexis forceps is used via 'open sky'. Delivery of the nucleus is achieved via 'open sky' by means of manual irrigation, and removal of the lens cortex by automated irrigation-aspiration.

The major advantage of the triple procedure is the faster visual rehabilitation and less effort for the mostly elderly patients. In cases of large deviations from target refraction, toric sulcus add-on posterior chamber intraocular lenses can be implanted secondarily to minimize the refractive disadvantages of this procedure. In contrast, sequential cataract surgery has the potential of a simultaneous reduction of corneal astigmatism (appropriate location of the incision, simultaneous refractive keratotomies or implantation of a toric posterior chamber intraocular lens). Disadvantages may include the loss of graft endothelial cells and the theoretically increased risk of immunologic allograft reactions. After the triple procedure, major deviations from target refraction have been reported. Since suture removal after PKP may result in major individual changes of the corneal curvature, intraocular lens power calculation for the sequential approach requires all sutures to be removed at the time of cataract surgery [91–93].

In case of cornea guttata without corneal decompensation, a clinically significant cataract may be operated on during protection of the endothelium by a dispersive viscoelastic agent without simultaneous keratoplasty after extensive counseling of the patient.

In conclusion, the postulated better prediction of refraction after sequential keratoplasty and cataract surgery is opposed by a markedly delayed visual rehabilitation. Thus, we consider the triple procedure including cataract extraction via 'open sky' under general anesthesia as the method of choice for combined corneal and lens opacities in elderly patients [93].

Conclusions

Corneal dystrophies require stage-related therapy. To ensure stage-related therapy, adequate classification with respect to histological findings is indispensable. Excimer laser PTK is the treatment option of first choice in superficial corneal dystrophies. However, proper case selection is of paramount importance. In a properly selected and well-counseled patient, PTK can significantly improve vision and quality of life avoiding or at least postponing the need for corneal transplantation. In case of deep stromal deposits sparing the endothelium and Descemet's membrane DALK may be effective. In case of endothelial dystrophies without stromal scars, DSAEK appears to be the procedure of first choice today. Still, there are some corneal dystrophies that require PKP on principle (e.g. macular dystrophy). Excimer laser trephination for PKP results in: (1) lower astigmatism; (2) higher regularity of topography, and (3) better visual acuity – especially in younger patients with keratoconus. Femtosecond laser application is the 'excitement of today' in corneal microsurgery. However, superiority of this high-price and difficult-to-maintain option is not yet proven! Minimal requirements for comparative studies between lamellar and penetrating techniques or between various types of trephination for PKP include (1) endothelial cell count; (2) rate of immune reactions (Kaplan-Meier); (3) BCVA and central power; (4) keratometric or topographic astigmatism (not only refractive cylinder!), and (5) a measure for surface regularity (e.g. surface regularity index/surface asymmetry index of the TMS system) – both with all sutures in and with all sutures out.

References

1 Seitz B, Langenbucher A: Phototherapeutic keratectomy in corneal dystrophies; in Reinhard T, Larkin F (eds): Essentials in Ophthalmology – Corneal and External Eye Disease. Berlin, Springer, 2007.

2 Hersh PS, Wagoner MD: Excimer Laser Surgery for Corneal Disorders. New York, Thieme, 1998.

3 Seitz B, Behrens A, Fischer M, et al: Morphometric analysis of deposits in granular and lattice corneal dystrophy: histopathologic implications for phototherapeutic keratectomy (o-PTK). Cornea 2004;23: 380–385.

4 Hafner A, Langenbucher A, Seitz B: Long-term results of phototherapeutic keratectomy with 193 nm excimer laser for macular corneal dystrophy. Am J Ophthalmol 2005;140:392–396.

5 Wagoner MD, Badr IA: Phototherapeutic keratectomy for macular corneal dystrophy. J Refract Surg 1999;15:481–484.

6 Dihn R, Rapauno CJ, Cohen EJ, et al: Recurrence of corneal dystrophy after excimer laser phototherapeutic keratectomy. Ophthalmology 1999;106: 1490–1497.

7 Lee ES, Kim EK: Surgical do's and don'ts of corneal dystrophies. Curr Opin Ophthalmol 2003;14: 186–191.

8 Pogorelov P, Langenbucher A, Kruse FE, Seitz B: Long-term results of phototherapeutic keratectomy for corneal map-dot-fingerprint dystrophy (Cogan-Guerry). Cornea 2006;25:774–777.

9 Das S, Langenbucher A, Seitz B: Excimer laser phototherapeutic keratectomy for granular and lattice corneal dystrophy: a comparative study. J Refract Surg 2005;21:727–731.

10 Nassaralla BA, Garbus J, McDonnell PJ: Phototherapeutic keratectomy for granular and lattice corneal dystrophies at 1.5 to 4 years. J Refract Surg 1996;12:795–800.

11 Auw-Haedrich C, Loeffler KU, Sundmacher R, et al: Characteristic distribution of deposits in recurrent granular corneal dystrophy. Ger J Ophthalmol 1996; 5:132–136.

12 Talamo JH, Steinert RF, Puliafito CA: Clinical strategies for excimer laser therapeutic keratectomy. Refract Corneal Surg 1992;8:319–324.

13 Das S, Seitz B: Recurrent corneal erosion syndrome. Surv Ophthalmol 2008;53:3–15.

14 Ferreira de Souza R, Kruse FE, Seitz B: Autologous serum for otherwise therapy resistant corneal epithelial defects – Prospective study on the first 70 eyes. Klin Monatsbl Augenheilkd 2001;218:720–726.

15 Reinhard T, Sundmacher R: Therapeutic strategies in recurrent erosion: mechanical trauma, epithelial basal membrane dystrophies, and idiopathic genesis. Ophthalmologe 2000;97:157–172.

16 Cavanaugh TB, Lind DM, Cutarelli PE, et al: Phototherapeutic keratectomy for recurrent erosion syndrome due to anterior basement membrane dystrophy. Ophthalmology 1999;106:971–976.

17 Seitz B, Langenbucher A, Hafner A, et al: Phototherapeutic keratectomy for recurrent corneal erosion syndrome (e-PTK). Report on 116 consecutive interventions. Ophthalmologe 2002;99: 703–708.

18 Das S, Langenbucher A, Pogorelov P, et al: Long-term outcome of excimer laser phototherapeutic keratectomy for treatment of Salzmann's nodular degeneration. J Cataract Refract Surg 2005:31: 1386–1391.

19 Wilson SE, Klyce SD: Quantitative descriptors of corneal topography. A clinical study. Arch Ophthalmol 1991;109:349–353.

20 Fagerholm P: Phototherapeutic keratectomy: 12 years of experience. Acta Ophthalmol Scand 2003; 81:19–32.

21 Rapuano CJ: Excimer laser phototherapeutic keratectomy: long-term results and practical considerations. Cornea 1997;16:151–157.

22 Szentmáry N, Langenbucher A, Hafner A, et al: Impact of phototherapeutic keratectomy on the outcome of subsequent penetrating keratoplasty in patients with stromal corneal dystrophies. Am J Ophthalmol 2004;137:301–307.

23 Kornmehl EW, Steinert RF, Puliafito CA: A comparative study of masking fluids for excimer laser phototherapeutic keratectomy. Arch Ophthalmol 1991;109:860–863.

24 Fasano AP, Moreira H, McDonnell PJ, et al: Excimer laser smoothing of a reproducible model of anterior corneal surface irregularity. Ophthalmology 1991; 98:1782–1785.

25 Szentmáry N, Seitz B, Langenbucher A, et al: Histologic and ultrastructural changes in corneas with granular and macular dystrophy after excimer laser phototherapeutic keratectomy. Cornea 2006; 25:257–263.

26 Marcon AS, Rapuano CJ: Excimer laser phototherapeutic keratectomy retreatment of anterior basement membrane dystrophy and Salzmann's nodular degeneration with topical mitomycin C. Cornea 2002;21:828–830.

27 Örndahl ML, Fagerholm PP: Treatment of corneal dystrophies with phototherapeutic keratectomy. J Refract Surg 1998;14:129–135.

28 Das S, Langenbucher A, Seitz B: Delayed healing of corneal epithelium after phototherapeutic keratectomy for lattice dystrophy. Cornea 2005;24:283–287.

29 Langenbucher A, Seitz B, Kus MM, et al: Topography-assisted correction of superficial irregularities of the cornea with the excimer laser. Klin Monatsbl Augenheilkd 1998;213:132–140.
30 Seitz B, Langenbucher A, Kus MM, et al: Experimental correction of irregular corneal astigmatism using topography-based flying-spot-mode excimer laser photoablation. Am J Ophthalmol 1998;125:252–256.
31 Epstein RJ, Jeffrey BR: Corneal graft rejection episode after excimer phototherapeutic keratectomy. Arch Ophthalmol 1994;112:157.
32 Hersh PS, Jordan AJ, Mayers M: Corneal graft rejection episode after excimer laser phototherapeutic keratectomy. Arch Ophthalmol 1993;111:735–736.
33 Alba M, Waring GO, Malaty A, et al: Increased corneal scarring after phototherapeutic keratectomy in Fuchs' corneal dystrophy. J Refract Surg 1997;13: 308–310.
34 Geerling G, Sekundo W: Phototherapeutic keratectomy – Undesirable effects, complications, and preventive strategies. Ophthalmologe 2006;103: 576–582.
35 Litwin KL, Moreira H, Ohadi C, et al: Changes in corneal curvature at different excimer laser ablative depths. Am J Ophthalmol 1991;111:383–384.
36 Dupps WJ, Roberts C: Effect of acute biomechanical changes on corneal curvature after photokeratectomy. J Refract Surg 2001;17:658–669.
37 Al-Rajhi A, Wagoner MD, Badr IA, et al: Bacterial keratitis following phototherapeutic keratectomy. J Refract Surg 1996;12:123–127.
38 Tervo T, Tuunanen T: Excimer laser and reactivation of herpes simplex keratitis. CLAO J 1994;20: 152–153, 157.
39 Vrabec MP, Durrie DS, Chase DS: Recurrence of herpes simplex after excimer laser keratectomy. Am J Ophthalmol 1992;114:96–97.
40 Seitz B, Rozsíval P, Feuermannova A, et al: Penetrating keratoplasty for iatrogenic keratoconus after repeat myopic laser in situ keratomileusis: histologic findings and literature review. J Cataract Refract Surg 2003;29:2217–2224.
41 Seitz B, Langenbucher A, Nguyen NX, et al: Underestimation of intraocular lens power for cataract surgery after myopic photorefractive keratectomy. Ophthalmology 1999;106:693–702.
42 Geerling G, Seitz B: Keratoplasty – A simple classification/terminology of current treatment options. Klin Monatsbl Augenheilkd 2005;222:612–614.
43 Anwar M, Teichmann KD: Big-bubble technique to bare Descemet's membrane in anterior lamellar keratoplasty. J Cataract Refract Surg 2002;28:398–403.
44 Hallermann W: Verschiedenes über Keratoplastik. Klin Monatsbl Augenheilkd 1959;135:252–259.
45 Fontana L, Parente G, Tassinari G: Clinical outcomes after deep anterior lamellar keratoplasty using the big-bubble technique in patients with keratoconus. Am J Ophthalmol 2007;143:117–124.
46 Richard JM, Paton D, Gasset AR: A comparison of penetrating keratoplasty and lamellar keratoplasty in the surgical management of keratoconus. Am J Ophthalmol 1978;86:807–811.
47 Lyons CJ, McCartney AC, Kirkness CM, et al: Granular dystrophy. Visual results and pattern of recurrence after lamellar or penetrating keratoplasty. Ophthalmology 1994;101:1812–1817.
48 Archila EA: Deep lamellar keratoplasty dissection of host tissue with intrastromal air injection. Cornea 1984–1985;3:217–218.
49 Anwar M: Technique in lamellar keratoplasty. Trans Ophthalmol Soc UK 1974;94:163–171.
50 Anwar M: Dissection technique in lamellar keratoplasty. Br J Ophthalmol 1972;56:711–713.
51 Sugita J, Kondo J: Deep lamellar keratoplasty with complete removal of pathological stroma for vision improvement. Br J Ophthalmol 1997;81:184–188.
52 Schor P, Rocha E, Cheema DP, Miller D: Calibration of trephine blade depth. J Refract Surg 1997;13: 89–90.
53 Shimmura S, Tsubota K: Deep anterior lamellar keratoplasty. Curr Opin Ophthalmol 2006;17: 349–355.
54 Anwar M, Teichmann KD: Deep lamellar keratoplasty: surgical techniques for anterior lamellar keratoplasty with and without baring of the Descemet's membrane. Cornea 2002;21:374–383.
55 Shimazaki J, Shimmura S, Ishioka M, Tsubota K: Randomized clinical trial of deep lamellar keratoplasty vs penetrating keratoplasty. Am J Ophthalmol 2002;134:159–165.
56 Melles GR, Lander F, Rietveld FJR, et al: A new surgical technique for deep stromal, anterior lamellar keratoplasty. Br J Ophthalmol 1999;83:327–333.
57 Marchini G, Mastropasqua L, Pedrotti E, et al: Deep lamellar keratoplasty by intracorneal dissection a prospective clinical and confocal microscopic study. Ophthalmology 2006;113:1289–1300.
58 Busin, M, Zambianchi L, Arffa RC: Microkeratome-assisted lamellar keratoplasty for the surgical treatment of keratoconus. Ophthalmology 2005;112: 987–997.
59 Yoo SH, Kymionis GD, Koreishi A, et al: Femtosecond laser-assisted sutureless anterior lamellar keratoplasty. Ophthalmology 2008;115: 1303–1307.
60 Ardjomand N, Hau S, McAlister J, et al: Quality of vision and graft thickness in deep anterior lamellar and penetrating corneal allografts. Am J Ophthalmol 2007;143:228–235.

61 Vajpayee RB, Tyagi J, Sharma N, et al: Deep anterior lamellar keratoplasty by big-bubble technique for treatment corneal stromal opacities. Am J Ophthalmol 2007;143:954–957.
62 Den S, Shimmura S, Tsubota K, Shimazaki J: Impact of the Descemet membrane perforation on surgical outcomes after deep lamellar keratoplasty. Am J Ophthalmol 2007;143:750–754.
63 Seitz B, Langenbucher A, Naumann GOH: Trephination in penetrating keratoplasty; in Reinhard T, Larkin F (eds): Essentials in Ophthalmology – Corneal and External Eye Disease. Berlin, Springer, 2006, pp 123–152.
64 Melles GRJ, Wijdh RHJ, Nieuwendaal CP: A technique to excise the Decemet membrane from a recipient cornea (descemetorhexis). Cornea 2004; 23:286–288.
65 Price MO, Price FW Jr: Endothelial cell loss after descemet stripping with endothelial keratoplasty: influencing factors and 2-year trend. Ophthalmology 2008;115:857–865.
66 Price MO, Price FW Jr: Descemet's stripping with endothelial keratoplasty: comparative outcomes with microkeratome-dissected and manually dissected donor tissue. Ophthalmology 2006;113: 1936–1942.
67 Melles GRJ, Ong TS, Ververs B, van der Wees J: Descemet membrane endothelial keratoplasty (DMEK). Cornea 2006;25:987–990.
68 Bahar I, Kaiserman I, McAllum P, Slomovic A, Rootman D: Comparison of posterior lamellar keratoplasty techniques to penetrating keratoplasty. Ophthalmology 2008;115:1525–1533.
69 Seitz B, Neuhann I, Neuhann T: Fuchs endothelial corneal dystrophy: current management. Contemp Ophthalmol 2009:8:1–8.
70 Koenig SB, Covert DJ, Dupps WJ Jr, Meisler DM: Visual acuity, refractive error, and endothelial cell density six months after descemet stripping and automated endothelial keratoplasty (DSAEK). Cornea 2007;26:670–674.
71 Holz HA, Meyer JJ, Espandar L, et al: Corneal profile analysis after Descemet stripping endothelial keratoplasty and its relationship to postoperative hyperopic shift. J Cataract Refract Surg 2008;34: 211–214.
72 Vajaranant TS, Price MO, Price FW, Wilensky JT, Edward DP: Intraocular pressure measurements following Descemet stripping endothelial keratoplasty. Am J Ophthalmol 2008;145:780–786.
73 Naumann GOH: Corneal transplantation in anterior segment diseases. The Bowman Lecture (Number 56). Part 2. Eye 1995;9:395–424.
74 Pineros O, Cohen EJ, Rapuano CJ, Laibson RP: Long-term results after penetrating keratoplasty for Fuchs' endothelial dystrophy. Arch Ophthalmol 1996;114:15–18.
75 Weiss JS, Moller HU, Lisch W, Kinoshita S, Aldave AJ, Belin MW, Kivela T, Busin M, Munier FL, Seitz B, Sutphin J, Bredrup C, Mannis MJ, Rapuano CJ, van Rij G, Kim EK, Klintworth GK: The IC3D classification of corneal dystrophies. Cornea 2008; 27(suppl 2):S1–S42.
76 Thompson RW Jr, Price MO, Bowers PJ, Price FW Jr: Long-term graft survival after penetrating keratoplasty. Ophthalmology 2003;110:1396–1402.
77 Langenbucher A, Seitz B, Nguyen NX, Naumann GOH: Graft endothelial cell loss after nonmechanical penetrating keratoplasty depends on diagnosis: a regression analysis. Graefes Arch Clin Exp Ophthalmol 2002;240:387–392.
78 Seitz B, Resch M, Schlötzer-Schrehardt U, Hofmann-Rummelt C, Sauer R, Kruse FE: Histopathology and ultrastructure of human corneas after amniotic membrane transplantation. Arch Ophthalmol 2006; 124:1487–1490.
79 Seitz B, Langenbucher A, Zagrada D, Budde W, Kus MM: Corneal dimensions in various types of corneal dystrophies and their effect on penetrating keratoplasty. Klin Monatsbl Augenheilkd 2000;217: 152–158.
80 Naumann GOH, Seitz B, Lang GK, Langenbucher A, Kus MM: 193 excimer laser trepanation in perforating keratoplasty. Report of 70 patients. Klin Monatsbl Augenheilkd 1993;203:252–261.
81 Seitz B, Langenbucher A, Kus MM, Küchle M, Naumann GOH: Nonmechanical corneal trephination with the excimer laser improves outcome after penetrating keratoplasty. Ophthalmology 1999;106: 1156–1165.
82 Seitz B, Langenbucher A, Nguyen NX, Kus MM, Küchle M, Naumann GOH: Results of the first 1000 consecutive elective nonmechanical keratoplasties with the excimer laser – A prospective study over more than 12 years. Ophthalmologe 2004;101: 478–488.
83 Behrens A, Seitz B, Küchle M, Langenbucher A, Kus MM, Rummelt C, Naumann GOH: 'Orientation teeth' in non-mechanical laser corneal trephination for penetrating keratopasty: 2.94 μm Er:YAG vs 193 nm ArF excimer laser. Br J Ophthalmol 1999;83: 1008–1012.
84 Langenbucher A, Seitz B, Kus MM, Vilchis E, Naumann GOH: Graft decentration in penetrating keratoplasty – Nonmechanical trephination with the excimer laser (193 nm) versus the motor trephine. Ophthalmic Surg Lasers 1998;29:106–113.

85 Szentmáry N, Langenbucher A, Kus MM, Naumann GOH, Seitz B: Elliptical nonmechanical corneal trephination: intraoperative complications and long-term outcome of 42 consecutive excimer laser penetrating keratoplasties. Cornea 2007;26: 414–420.
86 Seitz B, Langenbucher A, Küchle M, Naumann GOH: Impact of graft diameter on corneal power and the regularity of postkeratoplasty astigmatism before and after suture removal. Ophthalmology 2003;110:2162–2167.
87 Szentmáry N, Langenbucher A, Naumann GOH, Seitz B: Intra-individual variability of penetrating keratoplasty outcome after excimer laser versus motorized corneal trephination. J Refract Surg 2006; 22:804–810.
88 Seitz B, Brünner H, Viestenz A, Hofmann-Rummelt C, Schlötzer-Schrehardt U, Naumann GOH, Langenbucher A: Inverse mushroom-shaped nonmechanical penetrating keratoplasty using a femtosecond laser. Am J Ophthalmol 2005;139:941–944
89 Price FW, Price MO: Femtosecond laser shaped penetrating keratoplasty: one-year results utilizing a top-hat configuration. Am J Ophthalmol 2008;145: 210–214.
90 Steinert RF, Ignacio TS, Sarayba MA: 'Top hat'-shaped penetrating keratoplasty using the femtosecond laser. Am J Ophthalmol 2007;143:689–691.
91 Davis EA, Azar DT, Jakobs FM, Stark WJ: Refractive and keratometric results after the triple procedure. Experiences with early and late suture removal. Ophthalmology 1998;105:624–630.
92 Seitz B, Langenbucher A, Viestenz A, Dietrich T, Küchle M, Naumann GOH: Cataract and keratoplasty – Simultaneous or sequential surgery? Klin Monatsbl Augenheikd 2003;220:326–329.
93 Das S, Langenbucher A, Jacobi C, Nguyen N, Kruse FE, Naumann GOH, Seitz B: Long-term refractive and visual outcome after penetrating keratoplasty only versus the triple procedure in Fuchs' dystrophy. Graefes Arch Clin Exp Ophthalmol 2006;244: 1089–1095.

Berthold Seitz, MD, FEBO
Professor and Chairman
Department of Ophthalmology, University of Saarland
Kirrbergerstrasse 1, Building 22
DE–66424 Homburg/Saar (Germany)
Tel. +49 6841 162 2388, E-Mail berthold.seitz@uks.eu

Author Index

Subject Index